HOW TO SAVE YOUR TEETH & YOUR MONEY

HOW TO SAVE YOUR TEETH & YOUR MONEY

A Consumer's Guide to Better, Less Costly Dental Care

Melvin Denholtz, D.D.S.
& Elaine Denholtz

 VAN NOSTRAND REINHOLD COMPANY
NEW YORK   CINCINNATI   ATLANTA   DALLAS   SAN FRANCISCO
LONDON   TORONTO   MELBOURNE

Van Nostrand Reinhold Company Regional Offices:
New York   Cincinnati   Atlanta   Dallas   San Francisco

Van Nostrand Reinhold Company International Offices:
London   Toronto   Melbourne

Copyright © 1977 by Litton Educational Publishing, Inc.

Library of Congress Catalog Card Number: 77-2947
ISBN: 0-442-22080-4 cloth
       0-442-22081-2 paper

All rights reserved. No part of this work covered by the copryight hereon may be reproduced or used in any form or by any means — graphic, electronic, or mechanical, including photocopying, recording, taping, or information storage and retrieval systems — without permission of the publisher.

Manufactured in the United States of America

Published by Van Nostrand Reinhold Company
450 West 33rd Street, New York, N.Y. 10001

Published simultaneously in Canada by Van Nostrand Reinhold Ltd.

15 14 13 12 11 10 9 8 7 6 5 4 3 2

Library of Congress Cataloging in Publication Data

Denholtz, Melvin.
  How to save your teeth and your money.

  Includes index.
  1. Dentistry – Popular works. 2. Dental care.
3. Dental economics – United States. 4. Consumer education. I. Denholtz, Elaine, joint author.
II. Title.
RK61.D35   617.6   77-2947
ISBN 0-442-22080-4
ISBN 0-442-22081-2 pbk.

*To my mother
Lillian Sachs Grudin*

*"FOR THERE WAS NEVER YET
A PHILOSOPHER THAT COULD
ENDURE THE TOOTHACHE
PATIENTLY."*

> *......MUCH ADO ABOUT NOTHING*
> *Act V*
> *Scene I*
> *William Shakespeare*

Preface

This book really began 25 years ago, the first time someone came up to me at a cocktail party, flung back his head and asked, "Hey, Doc, what do you think of my new choppers? I paid $200 for them. Don't you think they're too white?"

For 25 years, I've been asked similar questions:

"How much should my daughter's braces cost?"
"Is it better to have a removable bridge or a permanent one?"
"Are gum treatments expensive?"
"Can I save money if I give my kids fluorides?"

At weddings, birthday parties, and wherever people gathered, invariably someone would come up to me and say: "Can I ask you a *dentist* question, Doc?"

The message was obvious and the idea jelled. Many people have legitimate questions about their teeth and the money they spend to take care of them. But they are either too embarrassed to ask their own dentist; or when they do ask, they get answers that do not satisfy them.

So I decided to team up with a professional writer, my wife Elaine, on a book that would answer the questions the average person wants to know. Thus, the title *How to Save Your Teeth and Your Money*. After all, everyone has *teeth* and everyone has a *wallet*. This book would tell people how to save *both*.

We used my experience treating private patients in my office and clinic patients in the Newark Beth Israel Hospital Dental Clinic. We also consulted other dentists and dental specialists in orthodontia, periodontia, prosthodontia, pedodontia, exodontia, and endodontia (Chapter 8). We investigated "extraction mills," dental insurance, and the mouthwashes and toothpastes you buy; and we wrote 51 letters to every state in the union (including Washington, D.C.) to determine how many dentists have had their licenses revoked.

Elaine played the devil's advocate, or, more correctly, the *consumer's advocate.* She took your part. She forced me to translate scientific jargon to understandable, everyday language. If I said "gingival mucosa," she would ask, "Do you mean the gums?" If I said "deciduous dentition," she would change it to "baby teeth." Elaine forced me to communicate at the patient's level and together we worked out *a comprehensive and practical guide for the dental consumer.* Unlike other books on dentistry, which are too technical to be of any use, we insisted that our book would talk plainly. And we would not dodge the one subject everyone really wants to know about: MONEY! We would explain costs, high and low fees, and payment plans; and we would spell out in dollars and cents *how to get better dental care for less money.*

THIS BOOK IS FOR YOU, THE DENTAL CONSUMER. It is a book we hope you will refer to over the years and pull out whenever a question crops up. It takes a humanistic approach advocating that patients are people, not teeth, and you are entitled to certain rights. You deserve information about what you are buying, and you should get your money's worth when you pay for dental care.

We think our book will help you do that. We think it will help you *save your teeth and your money.*

Melvin Denholtz, D.D.S.
Elaine Denholtz

Acknowledgments

The authors are grateful to a number of dentists and dental specialists who read sections of the manuscript and made suggestions and comments. They are: Dr. Bruce R. Barnhard, Dr. Noah Chivian, Dr. Lawrence Lieberman, Dr. Joseph Pollack, Dr. S. Stephen Rafel, Dr. Arnold A. Safirstein, and Dr. Michael G. Steinberg. These dentists were kind enough to review special areas of the book to offer written comments, to discuss the material in an interview session, and in one case to prepare a taped outline of suggestions. Dr. Bertram Kaswiner, Director of Dentistry, Newark Beth Israel Medical Center, took time out of his busy schedule to read and comment on the entire manuscript. For their professional expertise and excellent advice, we are grateful. We also appreciate the suggestions of oral hygienist Harriet Kushins and my dental assistant of many years, Gladys Grum.

Several libraries offered us valuable assistance in our research, providing data, magazine articles, books, photographs, and reprint materials of all kinds. They responded to hurried phone calls for this material almost on demand. They are: The American Dental Association Library, Block Drug Company Library, and The New Jersey College of Medicine and Dentistry Library.

And, of course, this book benefited from the support of our family — the writing and editorial skills of our dad, Maurice Grudin, and the encouragement of our children, Jeff, Steven, and Lisa.

Melvin Denholtz, D.D.S.
Elaine Denholtz

Contents

Preface / ix

Acknowledgments / xi

Chapters

1 "Whatever You Say, Doc." / 1

2 You're Entitled to Know / 5

3 How to Do a Dental Checkup on Your Dentist / 23

4 Dental Myths Exploded / 34

5 Check Your Dentist's Fees Against the Averages / 61

6 Tips on How to Preserve Your Teeth and Lower Your Dental Bills / 92

7 Dental Insurance Plans: How to Get the Most Out of Your Policy / 111

8 Taking the Mystery Out of "The Dontias" / 125

9 How to Get the Most for Your Money by Turning Your Dentist On / 192

10 When Money's No Object and You Want to Go First Class: Dentistry for the Rich and the Super Rich / 210

11 The Newest in Dentistry: Dentistry of the Future / 224

12 Dental Consumerism and You / 248

Index / 259

HOW TO SAVE YOUR TEETH & YOUR MONEY

1
"Whatever You Say, Doc."

Americans spend billions of dollars a year on their teeth. Yet few can tell the difference between a periodontist and an orthodontist. Dentistry, like diamonds, is a blind item.

Ask a father why he spent $1800 to straighten his daughter's teeth, and he will give you vague answers such as "I didn't want her to look like Bugs Bunny."; or "My wife said she needed it."; or "My dentist recommended an orthodontist."; or "Her teeth were crooked." As the TV commercial goes, "What's a poor father to do?" He wants to do right by his children, to give his family the best his wallet can afford. So he often lays out thousands of dollars without the vaguest notion of what he's paying for. "Look," he'll tell you, "what do I know? I have to trust the dentist and hope for the best."

Just as this father assumes, without questioning, that he's getting his dollar's worth, so do millions of people lay out billions of dollars every year without the foggiest notion as to the *specifics* of what their dentist is doing for them; whether they can get the same quality of dentistry for less money; whether the work is absolutely necessary or in their best interests; whether such work can be postponed without hardship or risk; or what alternate plans are available.

Far too many patients are reluctant to ask questions for fear of displaying ignorance, antagonizing their dentist, or other equally absurd reasons. Why? Their "reasons" will sound ridiculous. "I wouldn't want to question the integrity of my dentist, he'll think I don't trust him." "I'm embarrassed to ask questions." "I don't want to look dumb." "Frankly, I don't know *what* to ask." "My dentist's so busy, I don't get a chance to ask questions." There are many "reasons" the patient foregoes investigation, but of all the "reasons" the most common is, ... "What do I know? I have to put myself in his hands."

Not so! WRONG! WRONG! WRONG!

There is no reason whatsoever for a patient *not* to ask. He can! He should! He must!

Most dentists are honorable, well trained, decent men and women. They are *not* out to *get* the patient, to separate him from his pocketbook, to sell him unnecessary work, to run up a huge bill, or to do shoddy work. Most dentists are looking out for their patients and attempting to render the best professional dental health service possible. Most dentists sincerely consider the patient's ability to pay. They offer payment plans and suggest alternate ways for their patients to make extended payments. They are up to date, modern in outlook, and keenly aware of the newest scientific developments in their profession.

American dentistry ranks among the best in the world. Preventive dentistry, cosmetic dentistry, and restorative dentistry are all areas about which American dentists are unusually conscientious. Dentists often comb the literature, take new and advanced courses throughout their careers, and genuinely look out for the best interests of their patients. Today, modern dentists offer auxiliary medical care. They take blood pressures in their offices with a simple sphygmomanometer. They send out biopsy specimens to laboratories in cases where oral cancer may be suspected. They (or their auxiliary personnel) take time out to instruct patients in toothbrush technique, flossing, and plaque control that can be done at home.

George Washington's Wooden Teeth

Did you know that George Washington's false teeth were carved out of wood? Paul Revere, the man who warned that the British were coming, made Washington's teeth. He was a blacksmith, and blacksmiths were the craftsmen and artisans of that day. This crude set of teeth was held apart by small springs. Have you ever seen a picture of George Washington smiling?

Still, any patient who turns himself, herself, or her child over *without question* is foolish. Does a person buy a house or car through implicit trust in the seller, or does he do his homework and bone up on the subject? Would you fork over thousands of dollars on a virtually blind item? A man will spend hours checking out the frequency range for a new stereo system. He will check with salespeople, read consumer magazines and compare spec sheets. A woman will spend weeks combing the stores, investigating and comparison shopping a washing machine, dryer, or dishwasher. Yet both hesitate to find out, to ask, or to do their homework about *the one item they will be paying for all their lives: dental health care.* Parents will pay for their children's fluoride treatments, their daughter's orthodontia, their son's fillings, their own crowns, bridges, gum treatments, root canals, and perhaps eventually full upper and lower plates, *without ever knowing what they are paying for.*

This book will attempt to answer some of the most frequently asked questions or, at least those questions you *should* be asking. Why fill baby teeth? Can "buck teeth" be corrected without ugly bands and tremendous bills? Why does the orthodontist have to remove four healthy teeth on my child before he starts the work? What's a root canal? Why not pull the tooth and get it over? If I can't afford it, can I get the work done at a clinic? What dental insurance plans give the best dollar value? Can I put it off for a while? Is it going to hurt? How long will it take? Can I pay it off? Does pregnancy cause bad teeth? What can I do at home to save my teeth? Is my dentist a good one? Should I change dentists? Are X rays harmful? How can I save money on dental bills? What's the finest dentistry in the world, and what will it cost me? How should I select a dentist? Is that a fair fee? What's a dental implant, and does it work? Should I leave if the dentist keeps me waiting? Is gas better than a needle? How can I conquer anxiety and fear? How can I teach my child not to be afraid?

Don't go into the dentist's office like a sitting duck. Be informed. Be investigative. Be concerned. Also, be considerate. A busy dental office that is run well, is considerate of you and your time, so be considerate of your dentist's time. Don't plague your dentist with hostile, suspicious questions. Don't batter your dentist with lengthy discussions and make him go over areas he's already covered several times before. Don't badger your dentist with demanding scientific explanations that are not legitimately your concern. You don't have to know the melting point of gold to understand a crown. Your dentist is not obliged to give you a technical course in dentistry in twenty minutes.

BUT, do have a healthy respect for his professional training and ask for a clear, simple explanation of anything pertinent you don't understand. A patient who lets his dentist know he requires a brief, reasonable explanation will get better treatment and more thoughtful, respectful care than the one who says simply and docilely: "I'm turning myself over to you, Doc."; or "What do I know?"; or "Whatever you say, Doc." Such patients may get less than the best the dentist can give. Why? Perhaps, the dentist is apt to be a little bit more alert with the patient who is himself alert and on his toes.

You can be reasonable. You can be assertive. You can be respectful. You're paying for a service. You're paying for a *highly personal service done on your own body*. Like millions of other Americans, you are going to require dental care throughout your life. You're entitled to get what you pay for.

2
You're Entitled to Know

Ever watch a smart shopper in a supermarket sweep down the aisles selecting cans and packages for his cart? He looks, compares, evaluates. With prices soaring in today's economy, only a careless shopper randomly collects items without concern for value. The smart shopper compares brands for costs per ounce and grades of quality. He demands to receive a fair value for the money he hands over at the checkout counter. Why? Because he feels he's entitled. So are you!

You, the consumer of dental care, are no less entitled to value than the consumer at the supermarket. Going to seek a professional's services does not divest you of your right to know, to compare, and to obtain the best value for your dollar. You spend billions at the dentist every year. Yet for some unaccountable reasons, you feel stripped of your consumer power once you take a seat in the waiting room. WRONG! The only thing you will be stripped of, with this attitude, is your money. You're entitled to get the very best dollar value whether you're buying detergent or dental care. Remember, it all comes out of the same checkbook, and in today's marketplace, the value of your checkbook is rapidly shrinking. Don't add to your financial burdens by being a thoughtless dental consumer.

You don't need a disclosure of your dentist's class rank or his old test scores to determine whether or not you're getting your dollar's worth. All you need to do is to draw up a Bill of Rights for yourself, covering what you are rightfully entitled to. Then it's a simple matter of making some fair judgments about what you are paying for. Let's start at the beginning — before you open wide.

The Treatment Plan

You're entitled to know exactly what your dentist plans to do in your mouth. This is called "the treatment plan." It is similar to an architect's drawing of the house you are contracting to build. It's not an ironclad contract, but a plan, subject to modification (with your approval). It gives you insights about how your dentist intends to proceed, what work he'll do first, what the priorities are, and how he'll treat all your dental needs. You should clearly understand that plan, and you're entitled to a reasonable explanation of what the work entails. Here's where you can begin asking questions. At this stage you can make some good consumer judgments, but it is hopelessly ineffective to ask your dentist about that expensive gold inlay a month *after* he put it in. Once it's in your mouth, you're responsible for paying for it. So ask, understand, and discuss your questions at the treatment plan stage, *before* any work begins.

You'll also want to know approximately how many visits your work will involve, and how long the treatment will stretch out. Maybe all your work can be done in a few long visits and your dentist can see you in the evenings or on Saturdays, so you won't lose time from work. But, on the other hand, if the treatment plan involves months of visits (even years in the case of orthodontia), you should be aware of the personal adjustments you'll have to make. You may have to chauffeur your child to the dental office or incur additional expenses for baby sitters. Your time is valuable, too. You're entitled to consider the convenience of the treatment plan and how it affects your own life style.

Alternate Plan

You're entitled to know if there is an alternate plan and what the advantages and disadvantages of each plan are. Often there are several ways of approaching a dental problem. You're entitled to understand, through your dentist's explanation, what the alternatives are so you can weigh them and choose the best and least costly one for yourself. For example, let's say you have to have two teeth replaced. You're entitled to ask what's better for yourself, a removable or a fixed bridge. Of course the costs vary, but so do the relative merits of each, and you're entitled to pick the one that best suits you. Rarely is there one, and only one, right way to handle a dental problem. So pick the dentist who is not rigid, and is willing to explain and help you make a wise choice.

Results

You're entitled to know what the probable results will be. You don't want to be shocked when the work is done and then whimper, "But Doctor, that's not what I expected." No one wants to get turkey when he thinks he ordered steak.

"I wanted longer teeth," one man says *after* his dental plate is made. The statement, "I expected whiter teeth," doesn't serve any purpose once the work is done. Be realistic. Your dentist is not a magician. As an experienced professional, he can advise you; but questions of taste are simple, personal choices as long as they do not affect the wear and durability of the dental work. So know what the results will be, and talk it over before the work begins.

We all harbor unexpressed ideas of what we want and expect to receive. You're entitled to ask what is the reasonable "prognosis" (outcome) in your case. You may say that replacing those two missing teeth is simply a corrective device to help you chew better. But deep down, do you really expect your gall bladder condition to be dramatically improved, too? Do you expect the cosmetic results to be so overwhelmingly gorgeous that you will be swooped up by Hollywood? Do you anticipate such markedly clearer speech that you'll be awarded a promotion and raise? Be realistic. You're entitled to realistic results, not magic tricks. Don't expect the removal of your infected teeth to cure your backaches, make you look ten years younger, or improve your sex life. And any dentist who makes guarantees of wild promises is as suspect as the car salesman who swears your new station wagon will hum along trouble free for 50,000 miles.

However, you're entitled to know statistically how long a silver (amalgam) filling will probably last as compared to a gold filling. Then you can make a wiser consumer choice. For example, it hardly pays to crown your toddler's loose baby tooth (unless the kid just landed a million dollar TV commercial). You're entitled to get the results you expected, within realistic limits. Ask about the cosmetic results, too. Also ask about the cost of upkeep, maintenance, repair, and the psychological and digestive fringe benefits that lurk in your mind. Then you won't be disappointed.

Sometimes it can happen that your dentist's prognosis is too conservative and even he is astounded by the results. A New Jersey woman reported her hearing improved, and her nagging facial pain gone after her new dentures were made — a complete surprise to her dentist, and a delightful fringe benefit to her. But then no one ever complains about that!

Postponing Work

You're entitled to know what work can safely be postponed. You've just bought a new car (on payments); your wife needs an operation; and your washing machine just broke down. Sure you need dental work, too, but you're entitled to know if it can be done in stages. Ask: "Can we put that off, Doctor, without doing any damage?" or "Would it be okay to hold off on that crown 'til March?"

Some work can be put off, from a practical point of view, to a more propitious time when it will prove no hardship to you. So look out for yourself, and find out what can safely be postponed. Let's say, for example, your company is getting a dental health insurance plan in a few months and your work, or a large portion of it, will be covered by insurance. You've been thinking about having your missing tooth replaced because the adjacent teeth are drifting into the vacant space. Can you safely postpone the work another couple of months, or is it absolutely necessary to dig into your own personal funds and do it right away? You're entitled to discuss this aspect of your treatment plan with your dentist and to postpone that particular phase of your work if he advises you that a couple of months won't make an appreciable difference. It will to your wallet!

Or maybe you're getting a two week vacation next month and instead of taking time off from work for dental appointments (for which you're docked), you can safely put off the work and do it on your vacation (you weren't going away anyhow). Here again you're entitled to discuss postponement to a more propitious (profitable) time for you.

Free Choices

You're entitled to make free choices, unmarred by intimidation. You are the best judge of your own personal life and financial situation. Your dentist is the best judge of your dental situation. However, a happy compromise which is satisfactory to both parties can be reached if you clearly examine the alternatives. Sometimes you can get a dentist who "takes over" and makes choices that are properly yours. A seventy-five year old retired domestic wearing a partial upper plate (denture) had four teeth left. One broke. Because of her advanced years and her probably limited resources, her dentist told her he'd add a replacement tooth to her existing denture at a minimal cost: $12 for the extraction of the broken tooth, and $15 for the replacement. Total? A modest $27.

"Well, look," the woman hesitated, "couldja gimme a better job, Doc?"

"Hmmm...," the dentist demurred, unwilling to embarrass the "poor" old woman. "I can probably save your tooth through root canal and then crown it with a porcelain jacket. But that would run ... an awful lot more."

"How much, Doc?" she insisted.

"$125 for the root canal and $200 for the crown. That's $325."

"That's what I want!" her finger stabbed the air. "When I go through them pearly gates, I want that shiny crown tooth salutin' St. Peter!"

Free choice. She's entitled!

Discomfort

Okay. So you agree to your dentist's treatment plan. What else are you entitled to? You're entitled to know what pain or discomfort might occur. It's a sticky problem. What one person considers mild and expected "discomfort," another person might consider excruciating "pain." Your pain threshold is different from everyone else's, so no dentist can predict exactly what you're going to feel.

Sometimes a beefy 200 pounder feels faint at the first whirl of the drill, while a petite 90 pound octogenarian feels no pain. Who can tell? Still, you're entitled to know what pain *usually* occurs.

Ask. "Will there be much bleeding?" "Can I eat afterward?" "Will there be swelling after the extractions?" "Will my braces rub?" (Teenagers often harbor unexpressed psychological pain that they will look grotesque or cause discomfort when kissing.) "Will I lose time from my job?" "Will I feel up to driving home or should someone come along?"

You're entitled to know how long the recovery period is on extensive work and to plan your life accordingly. You're entitled to make choices based on how you might feel *after* the dental visit. Maybe you'll want to postpone that dinner party you were planning to give. Maybe you'll want to change that appointment for your job interview or the tennis tournament. If you have a good idea of what's in store, you can make plans with that in mind.

Costs

Now let's talk money. What are you entitled to? First and foremost, you're entitled to know BEFORE THE WORK IS STARTED what the costs will be. What is the projected minimum and maximum your work will cost you? Here you have to probe without flinching. You're entitled to know. Would you drop something into your shopping cart without an idea of the cost? Since dentists don't post their fees in their waiting rooms, you MUST ASK. Your dentist CAN give you a reasonable estimate. He can tell you what the probable costs will be and the range that your work falls into.

It's up to you to make sure there are no surprises (additional charges) at the end. The final visit is too late to cry out in righteous indignation that you were overcharged. But let's be fair. Your dentist may encounter additional work he did not genuinely expect. No dentist, however experienced, can predict with absolute accuracy the cost of your work — unless he builds in enough margin in the fee estimate to cover contingencies (an unconscionable hedge better called consistent overcharging). A filling can become complicated and turn into a root canal, an extraction, or a replacement.

Sometimes (rarely) the opposite occurs and your dentist finds his estimate was too high. The work went faster, it was easier than expected (you're an ideal patient), and the treatment plan required less time and visits than expected (as in a projected orthodontia case). Here you're entitled to ask if the fee based on eighteen months of treatment will be reduced since it turned out to require only twelve months. Don't expect a prorated reduction — that's pushing it.

Itemized Written Estimate

It's most important to get an itemized written estimate. A bill which states simply "For services rendered" is not satisfactory. It may all seem perfectly clear when you discuss fees at the first visit — all quite uncomplicated and easy to remember — but when you get home and try to explain it to your spouse, you may have forgotten. Even worse, by the time the work is completed and the bill slips into your mail box, your memory may not be accurate. You need something IN WRITING to refer to.

Take notes, too. Remember honest errors occur and human imperfections can be translated to a bill. If you have your dentist's written estimate that he charges $12 a filling, it's much easier to show that to his secretary than complain later, "But I *thought* he said $12." Some dentists prefer to give an estimate PLUS a contingency fee schedule to cover the root canal that might crop up or any other dental service not clearly spelled out. And remember, if you think you've been overcharged, don't hesitate to approach the Doctor or his secretary about a possible error.

Highly computerized billing systems can make atrocious mistakes, and busy group practices are increasingly employing such computerized "printouts" as bills. You're entitled to correct an error, request an explanation or adjustment, and expect your dentist to honor his written estimate. On the other hand, the patient who is outright hostile and convinced he's being fleeced doesn't get the best care. If you don't trust your dentist, change!

Payment Plans

Okay. You were billed properly and your dentist was accurate in his estimate. Now how will you pay for the work? You're entitled to know what payment plans are available and to arrange for payment in an acceptable way. You may notice that more and more dentists (and physicians) who formerly billed patients through the mail as a regular courtesy are putting signs in their waiting rooms:

DUE TO INCREASED COSTS OF BILLING, PATIENTS ARE REQUESTED TO PAY FOR THEIR COMPLETED WORK AT THE CONCLUSION OF EACH OFFICE VISIT.

Billing costs money and dunning with second and third notices of balances due costs even more, adding to the ever increasing costs of overhead. Who pays for these costs? You do, in higher fees! So prompt payment keeps fees down.

Nevertheless, you have a right to ask about deferred payment plans, alternate payment plans, pay-as-you-go payment plans, bank loans, or any other payment schedule that is mutually acceptable to you and your dentist. The patient who honestly admits he needs to pay off a large bill is more respected than the patient who proceeds with the work and does not pay his bill. Most dentists will try to find a way for you to pay your debts honorably. No dentist chooses to resort to the high costs of collection agencies or the added expenses of attorneys' fees. But he does want to receive what is rightfully due him. Therefore, it is wiser to admit you'd like to consider an alternate payment plan. You'll be respected for your integrity and you'll still get your dentist's best care. You're entitled to examine these payment plans with a full explanation of interest rates, penalty clauses, and surcharges so that you clearly understand which particular plan is to your benefit. There is nothing demeaning in choosing a payment plan. Get the facts and choose wisely.

Rising Costs of Health Care

The average American family spends about 10% of its income on health care, and the costs are rapidly spiraling. In 1975, money spent on health care hit $118.5 billion. Consumers tend to be less aware of rising health costs than food prices. The cost for dental care alone was 6 billion dollars.

Almost 25 million Americans are already covered by dental insurance. Maybe you have a private dental insurance plan. Maybe your company or employer carries a plan that covers your dental care. You're entitled to have your dentist (or the secretary) fill out those forms properly and help you get paid whatever is rightly due you, so that you receive the maximum benefits. You're entitled to this, but NOT to usurp the office's time unnecessarily. You can expedite the filling out of forms by writing in the personal data at home: Name, Address, Telephone, Social Security Number, etc., so as not to waste the dentist's time. You can be considerate in bringing any papers with you to the office instead of fumbling through a swollen wallet trying to locate your social security card stashed "somewhere" among the other things. Filling out a dental insurance form is a courtesy you're entitled to. But don't tie up your dentist's office trying to call your wife to find out your policy number.

Thorough Examination

You're entitled to a thorough examination. What does this mean? It doesn't mean pull the tooth out because it hurts and we'll worry about the consequences later. It doesn't mean a hurried, careless diagnosis without benefit of X rays, study models, or other diagnostic tools. A thorough exam covers many points and you're entitled to every one.

You're entitled to a *complete medical and dental history*. Here is where it's your responsibility to advise your dentist of any precautions to be taken for diabetes, hemophilia, allergies, etc. You're entitled to have *necessary X rays* taken as a diagnostic tool. If you paid $125 for a gold inlay, only to find the unX rayed tooth has an abscess underneath, you have a right to be mad. You're entitled to have *molds* (study models) made of your teeth whenever required so your dentist can reach an accurate diagnosis. This is true in cases such as fixed and removable bridges, orthodontic treatment, and in many cases where your occlusion (bite) has to be corrected. You're entitled to a thorough *visual examination of the teeth,* including air drying, which enables your dentist to get a more accurate look. He will then explore for poor margins, loose caps, faulty fillings, cavities, etc. You're entitled to have your dentist check your *jaw joint* and your *bite;* also your *entire mouth,* cheeks, palate and tongue should be examined for sore spots, irritations or tumors. Your *gums* also should be examined, with a probe, for pocket formations, color, and texture.

A thorough examination takes time to cover these items, and you're entitled to it.

Conservative Treatment

You're entitled to a dentist who is NOT fast to decide on an extraction. The best dentists usually choose the most conservative, palliative treatment and make every effort to save a tooth. Here's a letter to a newspaper advice column:

> I don't have much to laugh about these days, but when I do laugh, my uppers fall down. I'd give my right arm to have my own teeth back again. A good dentist can do a lot to save natural teeth. Mine didn't even try. He said, 'You'll be better off with dentures. They're cheaper, too.'

At first it may seem more economical to remove a tooth than to go to the expense of saving it, but that's penny wise and pound foolish. Sure root canal work will cost you more money, but the very best bargain, as this letter writer learned, is to hold on to your own teeth. There is absolutely no replacement that can substitute for your own teeth. Imagine the best artificial leg. Would you prefer it to your own even with varicose veins, ingrown toenails, and fallen arches! Besides, the cost of replacement can exceed the cost of saving the tooth. You're entitled to explore every possible means of saving your teeth and you're entitled to a dentist who is NOT extraction oriented.

Unnecessary Extractions

The Pennsylvania Insurance Department Guide reports that, "probably 6,000,000 teeth are removed each year that should have been saved through other treatment." Don't let one of those teeth be yours.

There are some places called "extraction mills" which blatantly remove teeth at the slightest provocation. They make little effort to protect your own natural teeth and often promise miraculous cures (of arthritis, diabetes) once the "bad" teeth are out. RUN, do not walk to the nearest exit if you fall into their hands. These mills are unconscionable and flourish on the fears of the naive and misinformed, the poor and unsuspecting. Before your dentist extracts your tooth, you're entitled to know why he rejected other alternatives to save it. You're entitled to have the most *conservative* treatment tried first.

Let's say you have a deep cavity that has just touched a nerve. It hurts. You can't eat. So your first reaction is: "Take it out, Doc!" Right? Wrong! Perhaps your dentist can administer a nerve treatment (pulp cap) to save your tooth and also save you the cost of replacing it. Consider the costs. The pulp cap might run about $15. But the extraction and replacement could run $500. Even if that doesn't work and the pain persists, you still have another option: Root Canal. Cost? Perhaps $125. Should the cost of saving your tooth exceed the cost of removing it, you'd *still* be smarter to consider saving the tooth unless it's an unbearable financial hardship. Remember you're entitled to decide. It's your mouth. It's your money.

And don't forget, you're entitled to the *least* amount of X ray necessary for a proper diagnosis. Some dentists recommend *full mouth X rays* (18 exposures), once a year. Others, once every five years. Keep track to avoid overexposure. We're talking about full series X rays of the entire mouth, *not* the diagnostic X rays of a single tooth or the regular checkup X rays which consist of 2-6 exposures.

Preventive Dentistry

You're entitled to the dentist who is prevention oriented — the one who has kept up with the newest, most efficient ways to prevent dental disease. Today's informed health consumer is on his toes and aware of how he can prevent medical problems before they are overwhelming. Instead of idly waiting for the heart attack to strike, he considers the benefits of proper diet, nutrition, weight, and cholesterol. It's smarter to prevent disease than to fight it once it has gained a foothold. So choose a dentist who takes the time to instruct you on the best dental routine to follow: How to brush your teeth. How to use disclosing tablets (harmless dye that shows where food particles are lodged). How to use dental floss. Face it. You have to be your own dentist every single day of the year, and no dentist can transform a neglected, abused mouth into a radiant, beautiful smile without your cooperation.

The dentist who merely "fixes you up" when you come to his office is doing a patch job, and is wasting your time and money. That's no bargain. You're entitled to a demonstration of proper oral hygiene to observe every day at home. If you follow a good regime to loosen and remove plaque (the film formed by bacteria acting on food debris), you can help to reduce the decay and gum problems that afflict 95% of the population. Save money. Ask your dentist about toothbrushes, mouthwashes, electric brushes, water pics, and see if he's willing to discuss preventive dentistry with you. Just as you take your car in for regular maintenance tune-ups, it pays to learn how to be your own Preventive Dentist.

Your children should be given fluoride treatments and/or fluorides with vitamins to decrease cavities, and they, too, should be instructed at an early age to establish good dental hygiene patterns that they can carry faithfully into adulthood. Don't wait for the first toothache to "drag" your screaming child to the office. Make sure the first visit is a pleasant, no-trauma occasion to get acquainted.

And don't bristle if your dentist is insistent that you come in for a three or six month checkup. He's not drumming up business. More likely, he's prevention-oriented. Some dental offices employ a "recall system" in which patients are reminded by mail notices. Other offices have the secretary telephone to arrange a checkup appointment. In any case, it's a good idea to keep these appointments. Sometimes a $20 checkup can prevent a bill of $200 or $2,000 later on.

Personality

Have you ever bought an item you didn't exactly need because the salesperson was so very nice and helpful? Or have you deliberately *not* bought an item because the salesperson was rude, short tempered, or arrogant. We respond to people's personalities as much as the item or service we're buying. So try to select a dentist whose personality corresponds with your own.

Some patients like a warm, folksy approach where the dentist comes on like good old Dr. Marcus Welby — ever patient, all understanding — a sort of father image. So what if there's a bit of dust on the faded lampshade. At least he remembers all your kids' names and that Tommy's gerbil had babies last spring. You like him. You trust him. And you feel confident in his hands. Fine. That makes you a more cooperative and relaxed patient.

On the other hand, some patients can't stand the dentist who "wastes time talking." That kind of patient is convenience oriented, perhaps even making appointments on his own lunch hour. He's irritated by folksiness. He prefers the fast paced, efficiency oriented group practices where three or four dentists assisted by a battery of dental hygienists, secretaries, receptionists, and dental assistants work as a team to get patients in and out efficiently.

There are good dentists and bad dentists in both groups. But assuming you're getting the best in dental professionalism, it's wiser to select a dentist whose personality is in concert with your own. One word of warning. The all-business approach of some large offices does NOT mean you should settle for anything less than a humanistic approach. You are a person, not a dental chart or the abscess on the lower second bicuspid. And any dentist who forgets there is a person at the end of his drill — not a chart number! not an impaction! not a crown! — should be replaced with a dentist who understands the feelings of the patient he's treating. The humanistic dentist is always aware that each patient is a person with his own unique personality, preferences, temperament, fears and anxieties. To ignore these and group all patients into "cases" is neither professional nor humane. The TV Medical Shows may refer to a patient as "the bleeding ulcer in 202" or "the cardiac arrest in Intensive Care," but you deserve better. You are a person with a name. Don't settle for less.

Every dental office has a personality of its own, too. Choose one that pleases you. Some offices are as awesome as Madison Avenue steel and glass towers. Others are small, shabby living rooms, so decide what makes you comfortable, relaxed, and at ease. Pick the dentist whose personality pleases you. You'll be more confident and relaxed.

Private Consultation

You're entitled to a private, unhurried consultation. This usually occurs before the start of the treatment. But if there's something on your mind that you do NOT want to talk about in the dental chair, you're entitled to speak to your dentist in his private office with the door closed. Maybe you want to ask some "silly questions," or "embarrassing questions," and you don't want the dental assistant to hear. Maybe you were up all night burdened by nagging worries. You have a right to dispel them.

Ann Landers, the syndicated columnist, reports "a woman was reluctant to have her teeth extracted because she was afraid it would interfere with her love life." Silly? Not to her! Feel free to ask:

"That sore on my lip, Doctor. Could it be a communicable disease from — kissing?"

"Can you get 'trench mouth' from drinking from the same glass?"

"I'm scared of cancer. This cold sore — could it turn into cancer?"

"Doctor, you think you could send the bill for this crown to my office? My husband worries a lot about money so he doesn't have to know about this. Okay?"

"I'm so scared, Doc. Is there a way I could go to the hospital and have all my work done while I'm asleep?"

"Look, Doctor, I can't afford it. Even if I pay it off, I can't afford it. Is there a free clinic that could do it for me?"

Even if you think your questions are "dumb," you have a right to ask them privately.

If your dentist has given you a long, complicated explanation, and you *still* don't understand (say it involves crowns, periodontal treatments, bridges and root canal work) ask *again* for a simpler explanation. Some dentists speak dental jargon that is understandable only to other dentists. They're not good communicators and they forget that the average lay person is not familiar with their professional terminology. Ask for a simpler explanation until you do understand. Use your own words and don't be defensive. You're entitled to understand what's happening in your mouth and what you're paying for. Maybe your dentist has visual aids, charts, or color slides which can clear up the whole problem. Maybe he can draw you a picture. Don't be ashamed to ask him to if it will help. You're entitled to understand. So ask.

"What's a root canal?"
"How does it work?"
"What do you mean my periodontal tissue is resorbing? Does that mean my gums are shrinking?"

Insist on translations you can understand. There's nothing mysterious about dental care, nothing you can't understand. But don't expect a crash course in histology either! You're entitled to good work and if you know what you *should* be getting, you're more likely to get it. Don't settle for improper contact points where food will wedge, high spots that alter your bite, or dentures that slide around and cause sore spots so you can't eat. Understand what you're entitled to. Ask for it even if it requires a private consultation.

Referrals

Sometimes a dentist will run across a problem that he feels is beyond his capabilities, and he'll refer you to a specialist. OR he may want you to seek a consultation with another dentist to confirm his own diagnosis. A good dentist will arrange this referral as smoothly as possible. He will send your X rays and records and assist in any way he can. If your dentist wants you to seek another opinion or to be treated by a specialist, it doesn't mean he's not a good dentist. On the contrary, it probably means he knows his own capabilities and limitations and is looking out for your welfare. Respect that.

On the other hand, maybe *you* initiate the decision to seek another opinion. Maybe you're dissatisfied with what's going on (it's better to talk it out than go off in a huff). Or maybe you're just not sure and want to get another opinion before you decide to proceed. You're entitled to the same consideration and cooperation from your dentist, just as if he suggested the referral. Your desire to seek another opinion does not imply that your dentist is incompetent and he should gladly offer his assistance. Ask him for the names of several dentists. You'll feel better if you get several names to be sure he's not sending you off to his golf partner.

Efficiency

You're entitled to a dentist who knows how to run his office efficiently. Today, about eighty percent of all dentists are in solo practice. The other twenty percent are in group practice, which means more than one dentist plus their assistants. You're entitled to a clean, efficient office that is considerate of your time. If you're still sitting in the waiting room an hour past your appointment or your dentist is constantly called away to talk on the telephone while he's working in your mouth, there's something wrong with the way he handles his work. Office appointments should be honored ON TIME, with reasonable latitude for emergencies, and patients who are matter-of-factly kept waiting over and over should demand better treatment. Ann Landers reports that one of her letter writers, infuriated because of time lost waiting, deducted his own hourly wage from the doctor's bill (Whether or not he got away with it, we don't know). Of course your dentist is neither a computer nor a robot, so be reasonable. But if you think you are being taken advantage of and not receiving the courtesies to which you're entitled, let your dentist know how you feel. He'll treat you better if he values you. And if he doesn't, you're in the wrong office.

Dental auxiliaries are the people who assist the dentist: the dental mechanic who follows the dentist's prescription for making restorations, bridges, crowns, etc.; the dental secretary or receptionist who answers the phone and makes appointments and does billing; the dental hygienist who cleans and polishes your teeth; and the dental assistant who attends the dentist at the chair when he is working on you. They, too, should treat you with courtesy and try to make your office visit pleasant.

Sometimes you get a rude, officious person who gives you a hard time and appears to be doing you a great favor to make or change an appointment. Don't accept that kind of treatment. As long as you behave courteously, you should demand the same from the dental assistants. They are there to help you, not to put obstacles in your path. Naturally, you will not endear yourself to the office secretary if you are a nuisance or permit your children to behave like pests. Don't expect to change appointments at the last minute, make outgoing phone calls, or miss appointments. You're entitled to courtesy, not pampering. But look out for the office assistant who is a Napoleon in white nylon, a tyrant exerting power over every patient. She's the one who says, "You're Doctor's ten fifteen." When she calls you that, correct her firmly with a smile and tell her, "You're mistaken. I'm not ten fifteen. I'm Margaret Kingley." She'll get the message.

Some patients feel cheated if anyone other than their dentist touches their mouth. "Oh, no. I'm paying the dentist and I want HIM to do it," they insist the moment the dental hygienist starts the prophylaxis (cleaning). This is, perhaps, a breakdown in communication more than anything else. Busy, multi-chair offices employ highly trained personnel who have passed state board examinations and are licensed to perform certain limited procedures in the mouth, such as cleaning and X rays. More and more states are recognizing the important contribution of trained auxiliaries in the dental health care package. Just as teacher's assistants help teachers to perform a better job, and secretaries type their boss's letters, a properly trained dental hygienist is the right person to clean your teeth and instruct you on proper home care. Insisting, "I only want the dentist to do it," doesn't serve you. In many cases, the dental hygienist gives a better "prophy" than the busy dentist. Remember she is expert at doing that one procedure, and she is working always *under the supervision of the dentist.*

Emergencies

You're entitled to emergency treatment when you need it. That means your dentist should see you if you are in severe pain. Obviously, if the pain's been there nagging at you for two weeks and you just haven't gotten around to it, you can't expect any sympathy. But if you're suddenly stricken with intense pain, your dentist should see you even if he's booked that day. If he cares about you, he'll "work you in" and relieve your pain.

Suppose you get a toothache on Saturday night or Sunday. If you can safely take a couple of aspirin for relief, fine. Then call on Monday. But there's no need to be a martyr if you're really suffering. You're entitled to a dentist who clearly makes arrangements for emergency treatment at times when his office is *not* open. He should provide either a "covering doctor" who will see you, or he should arrange for his telephone answering service to phone him so he can call back. The same is true if he's away on vacation. A dentist who leaves you stranded is not giving you the service you deserve. If he's away on vacation and you happen to get a toothache, you can't wait two weeks for him to come home. And a strange dentist is not likely to open his office for you on a Sunday. (You may have to go to the dental clinic of a large hospital.) So make sure you know how to reach your dentist in an emergency and what arrangements he makes. A 3 A.M. call will not win you Brownie points, so be certain your call is prompted ONLY by a severe emergency that requires immediate attention.

• • • • •

A good dentist is NOT threatened by a knowledgeable, alert patient. On the contrary, the patient who is aware of what he's entitled to is probably going to get it. That means you'll be getting what you're paying for, and not anything less. The *Sunday Star Ledger's* column "The Medical Consumer" reports:

> Too many doctors that we have come in contact with or heard about, prefer passive patients. Passive patients, after all, are faster and easier to get in and out of a busy doctor's office.

They also make more money for the doctor. Make money for yourself. Get what you're paying for. You're entitled!

3
How to Do a Dental Checkup on Your Dentist

Once a dentist has graduated from dental school, passed the State Board Examinations, and received his license to practice, he may begin to accept patients. Thereafter, there is virtually no effective way to check on his ability to perform. Having hung his license and diploma on the wall and unlocked his waiting room door, he is now authorized FOR LIFE to work in your mouth. Only on the rarest occasions is a dental license revoked. For example, Herbert S. Denenberg's *A Shoppers Guide to Dentistry* cites an amazing statistic. Of the 5,632 dentists practicing in the state of Pennsylvania through 1972, only one dentist lost his license to practice in the last five years. Obviously, there is hardly any accountability or meaningful reexamination of the profession.

What follows is a simple test you can administer to your own dentist. Do this dental checkup and see how your dentist scores. If he scores 4 or more, seriously consider looking for a new dentist. *Rip out the sheet at the end of this book and take it with you on your next dental visit.*

☐ 1. *Your dentist does not take any X rays.*

You visit a dentist for the first time. He examines you, but does *not* take *any* X rays, nor does he inquire if you recently had an X ray series taken by your former dentist. Failure to use X rays as a diagnostic tool can cost you, the patient, considerable expenses later on and result in improper dental treatment. It is almost impossible to practice first-rate dentistry without any X ray at all. There is no way to know what is happening under existing fillings, in between the teeth, or at the root end of a tooth. Without an X ray, it is possible for a dentist to fill a tooth that is already abscessed — the wrong treatment. Therefore, expensive and complicated dentistry can be avoided if proper diagnosis is determined through early detection by X ray.

There are several exceptions to this general rule:

a. A pregnant woman should not have any dental X rays unless it is absolutely necessary, and then *only* of the single tooth in question. The full dental X ray series can usually be postponed until after the baby has been delivered.
b. A patient with a history of radiation treatment or much medical X ray diagnosis should be subjected to the most minimum exposure.

It is generally agreed that some form of dental checkup X rays should be taken at least once a year, and a full series dental X ray examination performed every three to five years.

If your dentist does not take any X rays, score 1 point.

☐ 2. *Your dentist does take X rays, but he holds them with his own finger.*

This technique of taking X rays is extremely rare. It hardly seems possible that such poor technique can still be practiced, yet it persists in a few isolated dental offices. A dentist who uses his own finger to routinely hold X ray film in position is exposing that finger to periodic radiation, and cancer of his finger may result.

If your dentist routinely holds the X ray film with his own finger, score this item 1 point.

☐ 3. *Your dentist takes X rays, but asks you, the patient, to hold the film with your finger.*

This is a fairly common practice in many offices throughout the country. However, there are better techniques to use today. There are specially designed plastic holders that receive the X ray film, and the patient simply has to bite on the X ray holder to properly position the film in his mouth. Not only is this technique safer, but it generally produces an X ray of superior quality, in that the X ray film is not distorted by finger pressure. If you're wondering if you can get cancer of the finger from a single or occasional X ray, don't worry. It is virtually impossible.

If your dentist asks you to hold the X ray with your own finger, score ½ point.

☐ 4. **Your dentist takes X rays, but he does not drape a protective lead bib over your body.**

Not all dentists routinely use a lead bib. Estimates indicate that about one-quarter of dentists use it. New modern X ray machines that meet state and federal standards are designed in such a way that the X ray machine head itself is leaded. Consequently, very little stray radiation can leak from the machine.

However, the extra protection of the lead bib draped over the patient from neck to knees is an extra precaution. The dentist who routinely uses the lead bib for his patients is one who is extremely concerned and is taking every precaution. It is far better technique to use the protective bib.

If your dentist does not use a lead bib, score ½ point.

☐ 5. **Your dentist does not give a detailed explanation of his fees before the work is started.**

No consumer would purchase a large, expensive item for his home without a definite understanding of the price. Yet the dental patient may submit meekly to high cost dental work without any specific knowledge of the final fee. Why? "I'm embarrassed to ask." is one reply, or "I just have to trust him." is another. This is a foolhardy policy and can lead to angry recriminations when the bill arrives.

It makes for far better dentist-patient relationships if the patient has a full understanding of the work he's going to have done as well as *a written estimate* of the fee. This arrangement will avoid future misunderstandings.

Sometimes, when complicated mouth rehabilitation work is planned, the dentist can't be pinned down because he may run into unexpected additional work. This is reasonable. In such cases, a contingency fee and alternate treatment plan should be *spelled out*.

Avoid the dentist whose bills merely read "For Services Rendered." Avoid the dentist who is reluctant to discuss fees. Avoid the dentist who will not itemize his fees.

If your dentist does not give you a written estimate before work is started, score 1 point.

☐ 6. **Your dentist charges unusually high or unusually low fees.**

How can you determine if your dentist's fees are in line? You can ask a friend what he paid for similar dental work, but that's not always reliable. He may not wish to tell you the unvarnished truth, or the dental work he had done may not be the same as your own.

DON'T rejoice if the fee is very low. Few dentists are philanthropists. Your dentist may be cutting corners with substandard laboratory work (to lower his costs) or he may be short changing you in quality.

For example, he may be only pushing the filling in with his thumb instead of carefully packing and contouring the filling with proper margins and contact points. Quality dentistry takes time and therefore costs money.

Then how can you determine whether his fees are fair? Simple. Just turn to Chapter 5 which reveals the average fees, for the most common dental procedures. Now rate your dentist.

If your dentist charges unusually high or unusually low fees, score ½ point.

☐ 7. **Your dentist suggests an expensive treatment plan. You are undecided, confused, and wish to get another opinion. Your dentist is hostile, resentful, and uncooperative.**

Be wary of the dentist who discourages you from consulting another dentist or seeking another opinion. Avoid the dentist who is uncooperative about forwarding your X rays, study models, or other pertinent records.* No dentist knows everything! The professional person who is *not* afraid of a corroborating opinion does *not* become arrogant and angry when his patient wishes a consultation.

If your dentist pressures you to proceed with the work despite your misgivings, score him on this item. Comparison shopping or "dentist hopping" should be avoided, but if you sincerely are in doubt about your dentist's suggestion for treatment or payment, reassure yourself with a consulting opinion. You'll feel better about it even if you go back to your original dentist. And so will he!

If your dentist is hostile and uncooperative when you want a second opinion, score 1 point.

☐ 8. *Your dentist does not take a medical-dental history at your initial visit.*

Your dentist *should* take a proper medical-dental history in order to be aware of any drug allergies, heart condition, diabetes, or other systemic diseases. He should record the name of your physician for reference. There are certain dental procedures that are contraindicated if the patient has a particular dental-medical history. For example, if extractions were done on a hemophiliac (a bleeder) by a dentist who was unaware of that condition, grave consequences could result. With the proper history recorded, this patient could have been referred to a specialist trained and equipped for just such an emergency. If your dentist gives you a medical-dental history form to fill out on your initial visit, cooperate with him and be accurate in supplying this information. It is for your benefit and protection.

If your dentist takes no medical-dental history, score 1 point.

---

*Provided your bill is paid.

☐ 9. *Your dentist advises you that your headaches, backaches, sinusitis, diabetes, arthritis, and fatigue are coming from your infected teeth, and you should have them all removed.*

If your dentist promises that extracting *all your teeth* will cure whatever ails you, leave his office at once and seek another opinion.

It is possible, of course, that you may need several extractions. In fact, you may need *all your teeth extracted.* And certain facial pains and aches *can* be alleviated through proper dental treatment. But the promise of a cure-all for diabetes, arthritis, and even cancer, accompanied by the scare tactic that if you don't have your teeth extracted the condition will get worse, is an unconscionable tactic. It is imposed upon the uneducated and gullible to scare them to proceed with the dental work.

DENTISTS RARELY BEHAVE THIS WAY, PROMISING MIRACULOUS CURES. But an extremely small fringe group operates in any profession. So don't say, "Whatever you say, Doc." As farfetched and outrageous as this situation may seem, there are people in this country who acquiesced to such scare tactics and miraculous promises. They are wearing false teeth made at extraction-mills because they were duped by false promises. They still have the same medical problems, too. In fact these very problems may have worsened for lack of proper medical attention.

If your dentist promises that extracting all your teeth will cure your medical problems, score 4 points!

☐ 10. *Your dentist advises you that you need one or more teeth out. (No outrageous scare tactics or promises are made.)*

This may indeed be an excellent diagnosis. However, never automatically say, "Whatever you say, Doc." It is very easy to accept an extraction when your defenses are down. You're in great pain and you haven't slept all night. But *a toothache does not automatically mean the tooth should be extracted.* This is the time to ask the following questions:

- Can a gum specialist save this tooth?
- Can root canal therapy save this tooth? (Root canal therapy involves removal of the infected nerve and a high percentage of teeth can be saved this way.)
- Is there *any* way to save this tooth?

If you *still* have grave reservations that your dentist has not explored every method to save your tooth, don't be embarrassed to seek another opinion. It may cost more initially, but it can save you a great deal of money later on.

Caution: The patient who invariably seeks another opinion risks destroying a good dentist-patient rapport. Consider these exceptions.

- If you've been a long standing patient and have built up confidence over the years, accept your dentist's advice.
- If your dentist has cautioned you over the years that a particular tooth might need extraction, accept his opinion.
- If the tooth is a wisdom tooth or one that needs to be extracted for orthodontic purposes, accept his diagnosis.

If your dentist suggests an extraction without discussing ways to save your tooth, score 1 point.

☐ 11. *Your dentist does not see you as a person, but as a tooth.*

Here you have to rely on your own intuition. There are no hard and fast rules. However, ask yourself if your dentist is affirmative or negative in attitude? Is he psychologically aware of the need to put you at ease and reduce your anxiety? Is he a clock watcher who gives you the feeling you're being rushed? Does he give you his undivided attention, or does he interrupt your visit with phone calls to his stockbroker? Is there genuine warmth and caring on his part?

Dentists come in as many varieties as patients. Some patients like a strictly business like attitude, and others prefer a folksy chairside manner. Adjust your personality to your dentist's *and* separate his ability to perform from his personality. Unless his personality offends you, it's wise to overlook it in favor of good dentistry. The ability to perform high quality dentistry is not predicated on a great personality.

If your dentist's personality doesn't please you but his work does, score ½ point.

☐ 12. **Your dentist frequently keeps you waiting for an hour and is inconsiderate of your time.**

Any office can run behind on occasion. Emergencies arise where the dentist's schedule is interrupted to ease the pain of another patient, or attend an accident victim. However, consistent long waiting can indicate poor office administration, which may suggest that the dentistry performed is also poorly administered. *Remember, your time is also valuable.*

If you have taken the morning off from work to keep your dental appointment and then get a short, quickie visit, you are the loser. Add your lost time and lost wages to the doctor's fee, and your dentist may be too expensive. Ann Landers says that if you are kept waiting for hours on a regular basis, ". . . you have a legitimate complaint. Deduct your time loss from the doctor's bill . . ."

If your dentist makes appointments and then consistently keeps you waiting for hours, let him know your time is valuable, too, and score ½ point.

☐ 13. **Your dentist's office is unclean and shabby.**

The physical appearance of your dentist's office can be a good tip-off to his overall professional attitude. Since dentistry is very much concerned with hygiene, cleanliness, and surgical procedures, the dentist who puts a low premium on his own office's appearance does not set a good example. Any dentist who permits his office to remain unclean will incur a serious loss of confidence from his patients, because this suggests that his standards are not sufficiently high. Even if your dentist is so busy that he is unaware of such "details," his nurse, secretary or office personnel should correct these deficiencies. A consumer of any goods or services (from hospitals to beauty salons) deserves a high level of cleanliness and order. To accept less in a dental office is unreasonable.

Many modern offices today boast multi-chair group practices consisting of several dentists and many auxiliary personnel. Such offices are highly trafficked and see many patients daily. However, a busy office is no excuse. The same high standards of cleanliness must be maintained. Less than that should be unacceptable to you.

If your dentist's office is unclean and shabby, score ½ point.

☐ 14. **Your dentist does not employ any dental assistant or auxiliary personnel.**

Unless your dentist has four hands, he simply cannot practice efficiently and effectively entirely by himself. It is an impossibility to fill a tooth, develop an X ray, sterilize instruments, answer a telephone, take payments, make appointments, and perform intricate dental procedures without some help. Check to see if the assistant is out sick, on vacation, or has just stepped out for a moment.

The dentist who attempts to do everything himself invites constant interruptions. Unless he takes very few patients and they are long appointments, the dentist who is also the office secretary, receptionist, telephone-billing clerk, X ray technician, and hygienist has to be ineffective. A well staffed office with the dentist at the helm frees the dentist to concentrate wholly on YOU, your dental problems, and your dental health. Isn't that what you're paying for? So watch out for the jack-of-all-trades.

If your dentist works without any assistant, score ½ point.

☐ 15. **Your dentist administers a local anesthetic (a shot), but he does not use a disposable needle.**

Today, progressive, modern dentists rely on sterile disposable needles for the administration of local anesthetics. Each needle is individually prepackaged and sterilized. This guarantees that each needle is sharp, uncontaminated, and there is no chance of transmitting disease from one patient to another.

Before disposable needles were made available to dentists and physicians, cases of hepatitis were reported as a result of incomplete sterilization of a reusable needle. Why take such a risk when a foolproof method is available. True, it is more expensive for the dentist to use disposable needles than to sterilize and reuse the same needle over and over again. However, you can be sure that the dentist who accepts this additional expense is insuring YOUR safety. So don't be embarrassed to ask your dentist about this very important subject.

If your dentist does not use disposable needles, score 1 point.

At the end of this book, you will find a copy of this quiz GIVE YOUR DENTIST A DENTAL CHECKUP. Tear it out and take it with you on your next dental visit. See how your dentist rates.

GIVE YOUR DENTIST A DENTAL CHECKUP.
(If he scores 4 or more, consider changing dentists.)

1. ☐ YOUR DENTIST DOES NOT TAKE X RAYS. (Score 1 point.)
2. ☐ YOUR DENTIST DOES TAKE X RAYS, BUT HE HOLDS THEM WITH HIS OWN FINGER. (Score 1 point.)
3. ☐ YOUR DENTIST TAKES X RAYS, BUT ASKS YOU, THE PATIENT, TO HOLD THE FILM WITH YOUR FINGER. (Score ½ point.)
4. ☐ YOUR DENTIST TAKES X RAYS, BUT DOES NOT DRAPE A PROTECTIVE LEAD BIB OVER YOUR BODY. (Score ½ point.)
5. ☐ YOUR DENTIST DOES NOT GIVE A DETAILED EXPLANATION OF HIS FEES BEFORE WORK IS STARTED. (Score 1 point.)
6. ☐ YOUR DENTIST CHARGES UNUSUALLY HIGH OR UNUSUALLY LOW FEES. (Score ½ point.)
7. ☐ YOUR DENTIST SUGGESTS AN EXPENSIVE TREATMENT PLAN. YOU ARE UNDECIDED, CONFUSED, AND WISH TO GET ANOTHER OPINION. YOUR DENTIST IS HOSTILE, RESENTFUL AND UNCOOPERATIVE. (Score 1 point.)

HOW TO DO A DENTAL CHECKUP ON YOUR DENTIST   33

8. ☐ YOUR DENTIST DOES NOT TAKE A MEDICAL-DENTAL HISTORY AT YOUR INITIAL VISIT. (Score 1 point.)

9. ☐ YOUR DENTIST ADVISES YOU THAT YOUR HEADACHES, BACKACHES, SINUSITIS, DIABETES, ARTHRITIS, AND FATIGUE ARE COMING FROM YOUR INFECTED TEETH, AND YOU SHOULD HAVE THEM ALL REMOVED. (Score this 4 points and leave the office.)

10. ☐ YOUR DENTIST ADVISES YOU TO HAVE ONE OR MORE TEETH EXTRACTED WITHOUT TRYING TO SAVE THEM. (Don't include wisdom teeth or teeth to be removed for orthodontic purposes. Score 1 point.)

11. ☐ YOUR DENTIST DOES NOT SEE YOU AS A PERSON, BUT AS A TOOTH. (Score ½ point.)

12. ☐ YOUR DENTIST FREQUENTLY KEEPS YOU WAITING FOR AN HOUR, AND IS INCONSIDERATE OF YOUR TIME. (Score ½ point.)

13. ☐ YOUR DENTIST'S OFFICE IS UNCLEAN AND SHABBY. (Score ½ point.)

14. ☐ YOUR DENTIST DOES NOT EMPLOY ANY DENTAL ASSISTANT OR AUXILIARY PERSONNEL. (Score ½ point.)

15. ☐ YOUR DENTIST DOES NOT USE DISPOSABLE NEEDLES. (Score 1 point.)

☐ TOTAL SCORE

This dental checkup on your dentist is meant to be a guideline for you to make some sensible evaluations about your dentist and to decide if you are getting the dental services you are paying for. The more aware you are as a dental consumer, the better dentistry you are apt to receive. By administering this *DENTAL CHECKUP ON YOUR DENTIST* you are bound to get better quality dentistry and a more satisfactory dentist-patient relationship.
(You may want to show your dentist how he scored.)

4
Dental Myths Exploded

"How did I get this abscess?"
"Why are my teeth crooked?"
"What caused my gums to shrink?"

These are questions the modern dentist is obliged to answer because his patients confront him with them daily. Fortunately, your dentist has many scientific sources from which he can draw answers.

Although early civilizations did not have the scientific knowledge we have today, they too questioned the sources of human illnesses, the proper ways to protect themselves from bodily harm, and the most effective treatments for relief of pain. People have always wondered about these things. In seeking explanations for what they did not understand, they made up answers that seemed to them to be satisfactory. Sometimes they embellished, lacing their answers with stories and weaving anecdotes and fanciful dramas into them. Many of these, far fetched as they may seem to be, have come down to us today, persisting as myths. The Greeks, for example, constructed an elaborate system of Gods and godesses who lived remarkably human and complicated lives full of adventure, intrigue, and romance.

For some reason, misconceptions about our bodies — how to keep healthy, how to avoid sickness, how to treat diseases — are the misconceptions that die the hardest. Ask anyone how to cure hiccups, and you'll hear a dozen tried and true answers, guaranteed to bring results. "Stand on your head and drink a glass of water," someone will assure you. Another person, offering advice on how to get rid of a wart, will tell you, "Bury a piece of string in your backyard, and the wart will be gone in a week." Each one is convinced his advice works, in spite of no scientific evidence to support it.

The spectacular development of modern science and dentistry is the result of many thousands of years of scientific inquiry, and many civilizations have made important contributions to the high level of medical-dental sophistication we have come to expect. From as far back as earliest primitive cultures, people made use of different species of plants for magic and religious purposes, believing these plants had the power to ward off evil spirits and effect miraculous cures.

> **The Toothache Tree**
>
> *A tree, the Prickly Ash, is commonly called "the toothache tree," because chewing on its leaves is believed by some people to relieve a toothache. In the West Indies, some natives chew ginger root to soothe the pain. We don't recommend you stock up on either.*

From the Greek physician Hippocrates and the Roman physicians Celus and Galen, incorrect theories such as "the four humours" were intertwined with correct theories to form the basis of medical information. In the Middle Ages, herbs and plants were again commonly used, this time for medicinal purposes. And today digitalis, which is widely used for heart patients, owes a debt to early doctors who advocated its use long before they understood the pharmacological explanation for its effectiveness.

It was not until the Renaissance that medicine advanced dramatically, when, with the study of anatomy, it corrected many of the false ideas that were commonly accepted about the human body. With William Harvey's demonstration of the circulation of the blood, and with the development of basic concepts of the germ theory of disease, medical science engaged in a new path of exploration, taking a giant leap forward, and dispelling notions that diseases were the work of witches and devils.

Since 1800, the advancement of modern medicine has plunged ahead through basic ideas of antisepsis (which made surgical procedures safer), chemotherapy, microscopic diagnosis, X ray, antibiotics, vitamins, hormones, radioactive isotopes, immunization, lasers, organ transplants, and genetic engineering. As scientific knowledge offered us better explanations of the unknown, we no longer had to rely on myths and misconceptions. Laboratory experiments clearly demonstrated the rational basis of medical knowledge with the result that these misconceptions slowly eroded and were replaced by the indisputable evidence of science.

In spite of this proliferation of conclusive scientific documentation, there remains today a body of myths and misconceptions that hang on and are not easily dispelled. Although we like to profess how modern and up to date we are in our scientific attitudes, we still perpetuate a body of misconceptions about health. "Wear a clove of garlic around your neck and you'll stave off sickness." Scientific evidence? None. (Although no one will dispute the fact that wearing garlic will greatly reduce your number of close contacts.) It's interesting to observe here that misconceptions about the mouth, teeth, and gums abound, while misconceptions about the less visible organs such as the kidneys and liver are far less in number and emotional intensity.

Perhaps we can attribute the high incidence of dental myths to the fact that the mouth is the area of pleasure and gratification. From our earliest days of infancy, we associate the mouth with nourishment and oral gratification; later with the pleasure of chewing and swallowing, eating, drinking, kissing, speaking, and singing. Any interruption of these services is sharply felt.

Gets $275,000 for Lack of Kisses

For a Detroit housewife who can't feel a thing when she kisses her husband, the circuit court jury had more than sympathy. Clare Tomie was awarded $275,000 because part of a drill broke off during a dental operation and became embedded in her jaw. Result? She suffered permanent numbness in her lips.

A tiny canker sore the size of a pin head located on the lip or inside the cheek seems infinitely larger to us, both anatomically and psychologically, than its actual size. It distresses us far beyond its importance as a dental disease. Since so much daily usage and activity are focused around the mouth, it is not surprising to encounter many myths and misconceptions about its care and proper function.

After twenty-five years of clinical practice, here are some of the most common myths and misconceptions patients have expressed to me. Let's examine those that are most bandied about and see how they hold up scientifically. The dental consumer who is informed is less likely to be duped and more likely to get his money's worth. You've probably heard some of these. Perhaps you even believe a few yourself.

Pregnancy Causes Bad Teeth

"When I had my last baby, all my teeth went bad," the young mother declared.

Once and for all, let's put this myth to rest. Pregnancy does NOT cause teeth to decay, in spite of the fact that many women associate pregnancy with dental troubles.

It is easy to see where certain factors lead to this erroneous conclusion. The woman who is caught up in the excitement and planning for her new baby is likely to put off her own dental checkup during the busy months before her baby is born. She is buying the layette, furnishing the baby's room, and arranging adjustments in her home or job schedule, so it's convenient to put off her own regular six month checkup "until after the baby is born." Once the baby arrives she is even busier, so again she postpones her own dental visit. Instead of a six month lapse between office visits, the time may stretch to a year or two. Obviously, more dental work will be discovered in a time period of two years than a six month checkup.

To compound this situation still futher, the mother may be so preoccupied with the new baby and the demands of her new schedule that she neglects herself, her own dental hygiene, and her own nutritional needs. Her meals may be interrupted, even skipped. She may resort to nibbling junk food high in sweets and carbohydrates. Such a combination of poor nutrition and careless dental hygiene is bound to be dramatically revealed in her first visit "after the baby."

Of course, women experience certain hormonal changes during pregnancy, too. These changes may produce a temporary condition of puffiness or bleeding of the gums in the final stages of pregnancy and this, too, is often mistaken as evidence that "pregnancy causes bad teeth." Not so. Equally false is the notion that the baby robs the mother's teeth of calcium. The composition of adult teeth cannot be changed, once fully formed. Babies do NOT rob their mothers' teeth of calcium.

Your baby did NOT cause your teeth to decay. Maybe your stretch marks, your loss of hair, or your postpartum depression. But NOT dental decay.

It's Not Important to Fill Baby Teeth. They Fall Out Anyhow, So Why Waste Money Filling Them.

"I don't want to spend money on Billy's baby teeth," the boy's father told me. "He's only five, so I'll wait until he gets his permanent teeth before I have them filled."

Parents who follow that line of thinking are inviting trouble. Let's look at the facts. There are twenty deciduous teeth called "primary teeth" or "baby teeth." The earliest ones to erupt are the central incisors (front teeth), which appear around six months, and are followed by the other baby teeth until all twenty primary teeth have erupted by around twenty-four months. This schedule has latitude in it, and some babies may not get their first tooth until nine months, and their last primary tooth, the second molar, until twenty months. Some of these primary teeth are replaced at about six or seven years of age when the permanent teeth begin to come in. From then until about twelve to fourteen, all of the permanent teeth erupt, with the exception of the third molars. They usually arrive around eighteen to twenty-one and are commonly called "wisdom teeth."

Some people believe that since baby teeth fall out in a few years anyhow, it's foolish to spend money on them. False. The primary teeth perform many vital functions. Obviously, they help the child chew his food thoroughly. Primary teeth that are decayed or infected cannot do the proper job. The primary teeth also guide the permanent tooth buds into their proper position in the jaw bone. If a baby tooth is lost or extracted prematurely, it usually causes the adjacent teeth to drift into the extraction space. This can "lock out" the permanent tooth from its proper position. When the adjoining teeth drift into the space, other irregularities may result in the permanent teeth which can give rise to costly orthodontic problems later on. Therefore, the money spent on preserving the early deciduous teeth can avert the expenditure of large sums to reposition the permanent teeth at a later date. *You can avoid expensive orthodontic bills by taking care of your child's primary teeth as they need it.*

In addition to chewing and guiding the permanent tooth buds into position, the primary teeth function by contributing to the child's appearance and his facial expression. They are also his tools for correct speech. Some of the primary teeth may be kept until the child reaches twelve or thirteen and is in Junior High School. Therefore, it is important that they be maintained with the same degree of care as the permanent teeth.

It is also untrue that filling primary teeth can weaken the permanent teeth. On the contrary, an infected primary tooth may adversely effect the developing permanent tooth. In the event that a primary tooth has been extracted before the permanent tooth erupts, it is still not too late to guide the permanent tooth bud into place with a "space maintainer." This appliance reserves the space for the permanent tooth and prevents adjacent teeth from drifting, therefore avoiding orthodontic corrections or surgical procedures later on. Ask your dentist about a space maintainer if your child has lost a primary tooth prematurely. While it is not necessary in every case, you should discuss it with your dentist. It is in your child's best interests dentally, and yours economically, to consider it.

Filling a Primary Tooth is Easier Than an Adult Tooth, so the Dentist should Charge Less.

"You mean Billy's filling costs just as much as mine?" the incredulous father asked.

Some patients are surprised when they are charged just as much for having their child's tooth filled, as their own. They genuinely believe it is easier for the dentist, that it requires less filling material because the child's tooth is smaller, and it requires less time and skill. This is a misconception based on misinformation.

Many parents are also surprised when told their four or five year old has a cavity. Yet surveys have shown that 50% of two year olds have at least one decayed tooth.

The procedure in filling your child's primary tooth is basically the same one your dentist employs to fill your own permanent tooth. However, he must modify some aspects of the work according to the smaller size and shape of the primary tooth. As a matter of fact, it can be considerably more difficult to work in the smaller area of a child's mouth. It can be more tedious and exacting, too. The quality of the filling material must be every bit as good as the one used for your own permanent teeth.

Why is it more difficult to work on a child? Frequently a child will not offer the same degree of cooperation as an adult. It requires more skill to work on a child who is apprehensive, hostile, or crying. If the child is in pain, he may be jiggling around in the chair, fidgeting, or fighting the dentist. Children under stress have been known to grab the dentist's hand while he is drilling, and even bite him or land a few sharp kicks at their tormentor. On top of that, one yelp from Billy often brings an equally apprehensive mother flying in from the waiting room (if she's not already standing by), a situation more likely to create pandemonium than a relaxed cooperative venture.

Try to find a dentist who likes children and earns their respect by working well with them. But don't feel obliged to use the same dentist who works on your own teeth for your child. Different skills and different temperaments may be required. You may prefer to consult a dentist who works exclusively on children, a pedodontist. But don't overlook your own family dentist, who may work just as effectively on your child as on yourself. If your dentist agrees to treat your children, and you are satisfied with the arrangement, don't ask him, "Will you charge less for Billy's filling? It's only a baby tooth." *There's no short cut or cut rate dentistry in filling your child's primary tooth.*

Infected Teeth Cause Backaches, Arthritis and Bursitis.

"Pull the tooth, Doctor. I just know this nagging backache'll clear up once the tooth's out."

This patient, age 42 and perhaps twenty pounds overweight, was convinced his backache was caused by his infected tooth, and he wanted to have it extracted.

Over the years I have heard similar requests to have perfectly treatable teeth extracted when patients insist their backaches, arthritis, and overall fatigue are directly due to their teeth. They often urge me, "Pull it, Doctor, and all my troubles will be over."

It is true that years ago some dentists and physicians believed the theory that teeth were "a foci of infection," thereby causing systemic diseases. As a result of this flimsy theory, the wholesale extraction of teeth was a common procedure to relieve vague and undiagnosed pains. While it is true that tooth pain can be referred *locally* into the ear, the temporomandibular joint of the face, and the head, a bad tooth will NOT cause pain in a remote area of the body such as the bursa of a shoulder or the arthritic joint of a finger. The patient who asks, "Could my bursitis be caused by this tooth?" should be assured the answer is NO, that it is a misconception.

Sometimes a patient will report to me, with great satisfaction, "The day you took out that bad tooth my backache cleared up." Does that constitute proof? The question of cause and effect here is highly suspect. If this patient's tire blew out the day of a new moon, we are really stretching cause and effect to blame the moon for the blowout. In addition to the highly suspect logic, a patient who accepts as proof his temporary miraculous cure is badly served medically. What usually happens is that in a few weeks or months the temporary cure has faded and the pain recurs. Such tooth-extraction-cures merely mask the true nature of an illness and make medical diagnosis more difficult. Therefore, the patient who lays all the blame for his medical troubles on his teeth is merely postponing the proper medical attention he sorely needs. It is not only dangerous to delay medical attention, but it can be costly as well. Since early detection and attention may prevent the need for long and expensive medical treatments, the wise dental consumer will also seek proper care from a competent physician.

Of course, it is possible that digestive complaints can be caused by dental problems. Here it is easy to observe the relationship of the teeth to the digestive process because the teeth prepare the food for digestion through mastication. If your teeth do not meet properly, your biting and chewing processes are incomplete. This puts additional stress on the stomach and the digestive tract to complete the job your teeth failed to do. Another danger is that, if your teeth are missing, you may be "gumming" your food because you are uncomfortable. This may induce you to resort to a soft diet, eliminating fresh fruit, nuts, and meat. You can't bite into an apple or chew a steak. Such faulty diet inevitably leads to nutritional deficiencies which in turn can cause burdensome and severe health consequences. Here your dentist in consultation with your physician can work together to restore your health.

If you are a wise consumer, you are aware of this. *Don't neglect your medical problems by blaming it all on your teeth. That's a misconception.*

> **Don't Blame It on Your Teeth**
>
> *Most anginal pain is referred to the shoulders, arms, and neck. But researchers report that in 18% of all cardiac cases, the pain is referred only to the jaws and teeth. Your toothache could be straight from the heart.*

Headaches Can't Come From Your Teeth

"I've gone to two dentists, a specialist, a psychologist, and a physician, and these headaches are still driving me crazy," the 38 year old journalist complained. She was suffering from TMJ syndrome, an often overlooked disorder of the temporomandibular joint of the jaw.

What are the symptoms? Nagging headaches, pain in the ears, neck, and shoulders. In fact, the symptoms are so diverse and baffling, they can mimic migraine headaches, vertigo, ringing in the ears, sinus pains, hearing loss, and tic doulourex (a painful nervous disorder). Often, when the TMJ problem is not pinpointed, the patient's symptoms may be mistakenly attributed to psychological problems and the patient is referred to a psychiatrist for relief of pain. While there may indeed be some emotional basis for this pain stemming from stress, the nagging TMJ problem *can* come from your teeth. How?

The temporomandibular joint is the hinge at the side of the face where the lower jaw meets the skull. You can feel it if you place your fingers lightly in front of your ears and open and close your mouth. Feel that hinge? If that hinge doesn't work properly, *pain can result.* What causes TMJ pain? A bad bite (malocclusion) in *either* false teeth that don't mesh properly, *or* your own natural teeth that are in malocclusion. Improperly meshing teeth can cause muscle spasms which, in turn, may irritate the TMJ. Dr. Harold Gelb, director of the TMJ Clinic at the New York Eye and Ear Infirmary, feels that the pain felt by 20 million TMJ sufferers may be due to muscle contractions resulting in "tired mouth."

Is there any relief for these nagging and bizarre pains? There is no one universal cure for TMJ pain, but many sufferers do get relief. How? By trying one of the many treatments available. First, see your dentist and rule out the possibility of malocclusion, the most common cause. You may get relief once your teeth are placed in proper alignment. This is accomplished by reshaping your teeth so that they hit more evenly, thus balancing your bite — a procedure called "bite equilibration." Another treatment is to wear a "bite plate" (usually at night), a plastic appliance which fits over your teeth to prevent grinding. This cuts down on muscle spasms.

Other patients respond to moist heat, muscle relaxing drugs, or the injection of a small amount of local anesthetic into the joint. Even biofeedback techniques have been used to control stress. If all else fails, surgery to the TMJ may be indicated, but this should be considered as a last, desperate choice.

Can headaches come from your teeth? You bet! That headache could be in your mouth!

If Your Removable, Partial Denture* is Loose, Save Yourself a Dental Bill and Tighten the Clasp Yourself.

"My plate got loose, Doctor, and I just wanted to tighten the hook a little, so I bent it with my pliers," the high school teacher told me. Then, with embarrassment, he cupped his new partial denture in his open palm. "And the hook snapped," he added. "Can you put it together again?" Unfortunately, I could not.

There are many handy men and women who can fix a toaster, rewire a stereo, or lay a new linoleum floor. So it is understandable, when they attempt to repair their own dentures, that their incentive is to save money on a dental visit. Almost always, however, it results in further expense, time, and frustration.

You cannot equate health economy with household economy, and the only one who should adjust your denture is your denitst. Of course it is tempting to try to tighten a clasp that has loosened up a bit, particularly when your denture is riding up and down uncomfortably in your mouth. However, bending the metal without proper

---

*A removable, partial denture is a "prosthetic" (artificial) device that replaces one or more missing teeth and slips in and out of the patient's mouth easily.

instruments can render that denture totally useless. The metal clasp can snap, or the denture itself may become so distorted that the entire plate has to be remade. This means a replacement costing several hundred dollars.

It is far wiser and more economical to go back to your dentist for this simple, inexpensive adjustment. Perhaps a fee of $10 will save you the cost of remaking the entire denture, a fee of perhaps $300. *Only your dentist can properly fit, adjust, and modify your denture.* To attempt to save a $10 dental bill here is false economy.

You Wear Full Upper or Lower Dentures* Which have Loosened, Causing Sore Spots. Buy a Home Reline Kit, Reline Your Own Dentures, and Save a Big Dental Bill.

"My brother-in-law told me to reline my own dentures," the insurance salesman admitted. "He said I'd save a lot of money."

Do-it-yourself Kits offer all kinds of incentives to the economy minded, and householders find the kits work well and save them consumer dollars in home improvement, furniture repair, or plumbing. But dentistry is *not* the place. Patients who intend to save a dental bill with home reline kits generally end up with greater discomfort and irritation.

Why? What is a home reline kit? How does it work? Basically, a home reline kit costs about $20, and is purchased to reline a loose upper or lower denture which is sliding around, causing sore spots in the mouth. It consists of plastic sheets which you fit under your denture and you bite into place, molding the plastic sheet by pressure. Sound good? Easy? Inexpensive? Actually, because of their chemical makeup, these plastic sheets do not "cure" or harden properly and they remain semi-hard, unlike your dentist's "curing" procedure which involves a new impression which accurately reproduces the contours of your mouth. Your dentist's impressions are then sent to a dental laboratory where a technician carefully processes the new plastic material under heat and pressure, bonding it to the old denture. Cost? About $75 per denture, producing a rebuilt denture equally as long lasting and effective as the original. Of course, the

---

*A full upper or lower denture is a "prosthetic" (artificial) device used when ALL the upper or lower teeth are missing.

end result is far superior to the best home reline job which may produce new and different sore spots and damage to the surrounding tissue. In addition to that, the home relined dentures imbibe odors of the mouth, and often do not fit correctly, causing chronic sore spots which may be dangerous. So in the end they are uncomfortable, unclean, and ineffective. They may hurt, slide around, and smell bad, and the dental consumer who has paid his $20 will feel he threw his money out.

By all means go to your dentist to have a professional relining of your dentures. Since dentures often last five years (I have seen some lasting twenty years) the reline fee for this service divided by five years means about $15 a year for comfort and fit which assures you of eating, talking, and feeling right. That's spending your consumer dollars right, too!

If you are a persistent tinkerer, and you are also tempted to "rub off" a section of the plastic denture with your nail file or sandpaper, you are courting trouble again. *Any kind of adjustment, whether it is a complete relining or a simple modification, should be done by your dentist.* For a small fee, most dentists will perform this quickly and accurately. At the same time you will be getting a checkup of the surrounding tissue to avert other more complicated problems. Don't waste your dental dollars. Don't do it yourself.

It is also a misconception to think that once you have a full upper and lower denture you never have to go to the dentist again. You should have your mouth inspected periodically, not only for sore spots but for shrinkage of your gums and bone tissue. Often a simple denture adjustment, even in the absence of pain, will make you feel better, eat better, and look better. *Don't be an amateur dentist.*

Wisdom Teeth are Troublesome and Should be Extracted.

"I want all my wisdom teeth out before any trouble starts," the young graduate student told me.

Stories of impacted wisdom teeth, abscessed wisdom teeth, and painful wisdom teeth can provide lively tales at a cocktail party, but the facts most people believe are rarely accurate. Many people are fearful of wisdom teeth out of all proportion to the evidence, because when they are impacted or infected they tend to be extremely painful, and can cause referred pain into an ear, or the neck and the head. So "take them out before they kick up" seems a kind of preventive measure. Even dentists disagree about their attitudes in the case of wisdom teeth. What's it all about?

The wisdom teeth are actually the permanent third molars and are nicknamed "wisdom teeth" because they erupt around the age of adulthood (thus wisdom?) 18 to 21. They can be troublesome, but they should never be extracted without a specific reason. Because they are located so far back in the jaw, they may be more difficult to clean and so they tend to decay more easily. If they are badly formed, they also may be more prone to disease. People with small jaws may suffer from impacted wisdom teeth, while those with large jaws and small teeth have more room for them to erupt. They are part of your permanent set of teeth and complete the 32 you are intended to have. Therefore, they should NOT be extracted routinely.

Your wisdom teeth may be called upon to serve beyond the usual services of chewing your food and providing facial contours. If you have had posterior (back) teeth removed, such as molars, your wisdom teeth then become a valuable abutment serving as an anchor for one end of your fixed bridge*. Without this anchor, you can not have a fixed bridge made and your dentist will be obliged to make you a removable partial denture. Don't limit your choices by saying, "Take out my wisdom teeth, they're only going to give me trouble anyhow." With good hygiene, your wisdom teeth can serve you very well and be no more troublesome than your shiny front teeth. Because wisdom teeth are not as visible as front teeth when you smile, they tend to be neglected. However, like all your teeth, they need to be cared for properly and their value to you should not be underestimated. *Just like the wholesale removal of tonsils, you'd be ill advised to extract your wisdom teeth without good cause.*

Orthodontia is Only for Children.

"But Doctor," the attractive young actress protested, "braces are for kids! I can't wear those ugly metal braces and elastic bands."

---

*A fixed bridge is permanently cemented in by the dentist and cannot be removed by the patient.

People who believe only children can take advantage of the specialty called orthodontia are mistaken. While it is true that most irregularities in tooth position are detected and treated in children, adults too can reposition their teeth and correct malocclusion. This term means irregularities in the position of the teeth causing poor fit when biting and chewing. Adults who suffer with "buck teeth," protruding jaws, crowded teeth, and abnormal bites are all candidates for proper realignment of their teeth. Orthodontia may be performed to correct such conditions and improve your appearance even if you're past forty.

Many adults go through life hardly ever smiling. Or when they do smile, you may notice they turn slightly away or move one hand up to cover their unsightly smile. It is not difficult to spot the adult who rarely flashes a smile or who looks off to one side to avoid smiling. These people are ashamed of their teeth, but they do not have to go through life that way. Adult orthodontia can be practical and simple. With the advent of clear plastic brackets that are directly bonded to the teeth, and removable appliances that can come in and out of the mouth, these orthodontic procedures become even more desirable, eliminating unsightly metal bands and metal brackets. If you are an adult considering repositioning your teeth to improve your appearance, you can be sure you don't have to become a "brace face."

Many adults who consult their dentists are seeking a simple improvement in their appearance, perhaps an uncomplicated realignment of a single tooth which is rotated or protruding. They are not seeking the complete reconstruction of their mouth and they are not seeking perfection. If the objective is to straighten one or two teeth that are prominent, your dentist may assure you it is a simple and feasible procedure that can be accomplished in a shorter period of time than you expected. If you've heard stories of tremendously expensive treatments that go on and on for years, you may be fearful to inquire, maybe even embarrassed. Don't be. Sometimes a minor realignment will be just the improvement you are seeking. It can produce an overwhelming improvement in your appearance and an important psychological lift to your spirits.

Americans spend billions on hair preparations, beauty treatments, and fashions, but often feel it is vain to spend money to improve their smile. So they deny themselves the advantages of cosmetic orthodontia. A Detroit secretary admits, "I was always self conscious about my crooked teeth, but when I was younger there wasn't any money and then, when I was in my 20's, I was too vain to wear braces." Check with your dentist. Admit what your objective is, and don't be put off by jokes or snide remarks about "railroad tracks" and "zipper mouths." Senator Fitzgerald, Democratic majority leader of the Michigan senate, was 33 years old and six foot four and he didn't buy those fears. Don't be cowed! *Don't deny yourself a pleasing smile because you think you're too old. Orthodontia is NOT just for kids.*

A Severe Toothache is a Sure Sign that Your Tooth has to be Extracted.

"I know it has to come out, Doctor, because it kept me up the whole night," the secretary moaned, one hand against her cheek. She was mistaken.

The fact that you have a severe toothache does NOT mean your tooth must be extracted. Of course, you're more vulnerable at this point. You didn't get any sleep, you're under emotional stress, and your overwhelming concern is to get immediate relief of pain. Take-out-the-tooth-and-the-pain-will-stop seems reasonable at this point.

Do not let this set of circumstances pressure you into an unwise decision. It's smarter to ask your dentist if he can save the tooth. Ask about root canal therapy, a method in which the tooth nerve is removed and replaced with suitable filling. You'll still have your own tooth, but the pain will be gone. Perhaps your dentist will send you to an endodontist who specializes in root canal therapy. In the meantime, he'll see that you get relief from the pain.

Of course not every tooth can be saved, and sometimes extractions are unavoidable. Patients who have neglected their teeth for ten years and present a mouth full of rotted root tips may find their teeth are unsalvageable. Then extractions are the only alternative. But if you are dentally aware of your options, don't say, "Pull it out." Ask your dentist to relieve the pain first. Then you can calmly consider ways to save your tooth. Since extracted teeth should be replaced, an emotional decision to extract the tooth may cause you a burdensome replacement fee later on. It's far better dental economics to save your tooth and avoid complicated and expensive replacement costs in the future. *Remember, the severity of a toothache is no outright indication for extraction any more than a sharp abdominal pain is an outright indication for an appendectomy.*

> **Occupational Hazard: Deep Sea Divers Beware**
>
> *Divers who go down 500 yards or more can suffer "tooth explosions." The tremendous water pressure forces the helium from their air supply into the spaces in the tooth left by a loose filling. Result? When the diver is hauled up and decompressed, the tooth explodes as the gas is released. OW!*

Root Canals are Painful, Expensive and They Don't Work.

"I couldn't stand it," the handsome airline pilot told me. "A root canal is too painful and besides, they don't work, do they, Doctor?"

A great deal of unfavorable misconceptions have grown up around the subject of root canal therapy. Many patients associate intense pain with root canal work and are especially fearful of the treatments. This myth has sprung up because it is usually the tooth that has been painful *all along,* perhaps on and off for weeks or months, that is the candidate for a root canal. Hence pain and root canal work are closely linked in the patient's mind. Actually, root canal treatment is painless with modern anesthetics.

Root canal therapy is a standard phase of dentistry and there is nothing exotic or dramatic about it. If dental decay is neglected or a tooth receives a hard blow as in a car accident, the nerve, or "pulp," may die. However, that doesn't mean the tooth can't function or that it has to be extracted. Your own natural tooth, even one in which the nerve was removed, is superior to an artificial tooth and therefore every means should be exhausted to save it. A root canal may run as little as $50 to $75 for a single rooted tooth to as much as $275 for a three-rooted tooth, *but you still have your own tooth.* On the other hand, if the tooth is extracted you might have to lay out $500 to $700 for a fixed bridge. So save your tooth and your money.

It is true, of course, that not all dentists in general practice do root canal work. Ask your dentist if he does. If not, ask him to refer you to an endodontist, the specialist who limits his practice exclusively to root canals. Here the treatments may run higher, but it will cost less than a replacement and you'll still have your own natural tooth.

A tooth that has had successful root canal treatments can serve you as a good functioning tooth for many years and possibly for the balance of your life. The percentage of successful root treated teeth is very high. *Over 90 percent of teeth given these treatments will last as long as your own natural teeth.* That's pretty good odds. The economy minded dental consumer who considers root canal as one of his options is making *a wise investment.*

Chewing Gum is Bad for Your Teeth.

"I told you, Jimmy," the young mother scolded her eight year old, "all that chewing gum is ruining your teeth."

This misconception persists even in the cartoons of schoolteachers who punish their students for chewing gum. Since most chewing gums contain a certain amount of sugar, it seems logical to Jimmy's mother because she knows that sugar is certainly not beneficial to the boy's teeth. However, let's examine the facts.

Parents often complain that in spite of their best efforts their kids live on bubble gum and sweets. Of course that's harmful. Studies have demonstrated that a nutritious diet is essential in maintaining good teeth. But what you do NOT eat is almost as important in preventing tooth decay as what you do eat. Children and adults who constantly munch candy, cookies, and junk food are bathing their teeth in sugar, a fermentable carbohydrate, strongly inviting extensive damage through tooth decay. The bacteria that is always present in your mouth acts quickly to turn those sugars into acids that attack the enamel of your teeth. Few adults and even fewer children carry a toothbrush around with them, and brush after they have polished off a Baby Ruth. So the danger is there and there's no disputing it.

However, some dentists have come to believe that chewing gum is not all that bad, and in fact some benefits may be derived from it. Remember, the initial sweeteners remain in the mouth a relatively short period of time. After the sugary part has been "chewed out," the gum may act as a cleanser and detergent, and even give useful stimulation to the tissues of the gums. Of course, the chewing gums that contain no sugar have all these advantages and none of the disadvantages of decay producing sweetened gums. There are many on the market in a variety of flavors. So if you're absolutely unable to give up chewing gum, *try one of the sugarless brands.* Encourage your children to do the same by setting the example. *You won't be harming your teeth and you may even be doing them some good.*

The Clasps or Hooks of Partial Dentures will Rot the Teeth that Hold the Clasps.

"I wouldn't have a partial, Doctor, because I heard that they rot your teeth," the stockbroker asserted to me. Is he right?

It is true that the hooks on partial dentures can make the anchor teeth more susceptible to decay. However, being forewarned that this might occur is the key to preserving those teeth. Partial denture wearers should be extra careful with their oral hygiene. They should remove their partials often and clean around the end teeth and hooks carefully. If you wear a partial denture and observe better than average oral hygiene with visits to your dentist on a regular basis, *there is NO reason why the clasped teeth cannot approach the same longevity that your other teeth enjoy.*

Another possible consideration to explore with your dentist is crowning or "capping" the teeth that hold the clasps. The crown which covers your natural tooth will protect it so that the hooks will go around the crown material or fit into a precision made attachment built into the crown. This eliminates any contact with your own tooth. This procedure is not inexpensive and can run $200 per crown or more. But it can extend the life of your teeth for many years. Here you have to weigh the advantages against your own financial situation. But know your options. Then it's up to you.

Bleeding Gums are a Sure Sign You Have Pyorrhea and will Lose Your Teeth.

"The minute I saw my gums bleeding, I knew I had pyorrhea, and I'm scared," the postman in his fifties told me.

Is he doomed to lose all his teeth? Will he have to wear full upper and lower dentures? Not necessarily.

Bleeding gums are only a symptom that something is amiss. Like a simple headache, it may not be serious at all. Of course you should consult your dentist, but don't panic at the first sign of blood on your toothbrush. Bleeding gums do NOT mean the end of your teeth anymore than a headache means a brain tumor. If you notice that your gums are bleeding, it could be the result of something as simple as poor toothbrushing habits. In your efforts to be thorough, you may be brushing too hard or lacerating your gums with an old, frayed toothbrush. By all means consult your dentist, but don't feel your fate is sealed and you are doomed. *You may simply have gingivitis, an inflammation of the gums.* However, gingivitis left unchecked can lead to periodontitis, commonly called "pyorrhea," a considerably more serious condition. If you do not get proper dental treatments for pyorrhea, you may well lose your teeth.

Proper treatment of the gums, called periodontia, has advanced considerably in recent years, and is a specialty of dentistry that you should consider to extend the longevity of your teeth. Millions of healthy, functioning teeth have been needlessly lost because the supporting structures, the gums and bone, have deteriorated. Like wrinkles and greying hair, resorption of bones is a normal physiological process that comes with aging. But with periodontal treatments and proper home care you can delay it.

In the case of simple gingivitis, your own dentist can suggest effective measures to alleviate the bleeding and prevent plaque buildup along the gum lines. He will also check further to see if you have soft and tender gums, if pus exudes from the gum line on pressure, if "pockets"* exist, or if your teeth are loosening. Such signs might be evidence of the onset of pyorrhea, and he may suggest that you consult a periodontist, the specialist who limits his practice to diseases of the gums. Do NOT ignore this suggestion. Unless you receive effective periodontal treatments to combat this deterioration of the gums and bony support, some or even ALL of your teeth may be lost. Pyorrhea is the chief cause of loss of teeth after 35. But you can do something about it.

Although periodontal treatments are not inexpensive, they are well worth considering. Perhaps your own dentist can treat you.

---

*A pocket is a space between the tooth and the gum where food can be trapped.

Ask him first. If he agrees to treat you, it will probably cost less than a specialist. In any case, do everything you can to restore your gums. In that way you will be investing in the health of your own natural teeth.

A Tooth Knocked Out in an Accident Cannot be Saved.

The young woman's voice was frantic. "Jimmy just got his front tooth knocked out. The permanent one, the new one!" she wailed into the telephone.

"Do you have the tooth?" I asked.

"The tooth? Oh, I don't know. It's probably somewhere in the driveway where he fell off his bike." She paused. "You mean you want me to find the tooth?" she asked incredulously.

Many people believe the myth that a tooth which was knocked out is a tooth lost forever. They don't know that a tooth "knocked out clean" (in one piece) can be reimplanted. If your child has a tooth knocked out in an accident, don't throw that tooth away. Find the tooth and wrap it in a wet cloth. DON'T wash it off to clean it. Just take your child and the tooth to your dentist as quickly as possible. If your dentist doesn't have office hours, try to reach him at home and explain that your child needs emergency care at once. Don't hesitate and don't be bashful. This is a genuine emergency and you're entitled to call for immediate treatment.

The tooth CAN be saved if it is reimplanted rapidly. Your dentist will see that the socket is flushed and debrided, and will perform certain manipulations on the tooth before he reimplants it into your child's jaw. Under favorable conditions that very tooth which may have been lying on the sidewalk will reattach itself into the socket and function normally thereafter.

There are countless case histories where tooth reimplantation has been successful; and they are not limited to children's teeth only. However, the greatest chances for success are in those cases in which a child's tooth was knocked out clean, is in one piece with an unbroken root, and is reimplanted promptly. A single rooted front tooth, therefore, stands the best chance. A word of caution. Do NOT try to reinsert the tooth yourself. Your dentist must perform certain preparations for the reimplantation to work. He must perform a root canal on the tooth you have brought to him, flush the socket, and reinsert the tooth. Finally, with fine wires he must reestablish it back in the jaw. You may forfeit any chance of success if you try to bypass your dentist. This is not the time to try to save money.

Fluoride is a Dangerous, Poisonous Substance Which Can Cause Many Harmful Effects.

"I've heard terrible stories about fluoride, Doctor, Could it harm my children?" a concerned father asked me.

The battle over fluoridation of drinking water has raged for years with both the pro and con sides making extensive claims. Those for fluoridation claim that measurable decreases in dental cavities occur among children, in areas where the drinking water was fluoridated. Those against fluoridation level charges that it causes a variety of psychological and physical diseases such as cancer, kidney damage, mongolism, allergies, bone damage, and mental illness. They point to the fact that a high concentration of fluoride is found in some rat poisons and insecticides, and conclude that this is proof that fluoride is a dangerous poison.

Like fluoride, there are many substances which are beneficial when taken in the proper dosages and harmful when taken in larger amounts. The trace elements found in multivitamin tablets, for example, are recommended in low levels because they are necessary for human nutrition and beneficial to our health. In larger dosages, they may indeed prove fatal. Studies show that fluoride in one part per million (ppm) in drinking water, effectively reduces dental caries among children. *Cities with fluoridated water like Grand Rapids, Michigan and Newburgh, New York report reduced incidence of tooth decay with no harmful effects.* Except for cases of dental fluorosis, commonly called "mottled enamel," there is no evidence of danger. Moreover, these mottled enamel cases occurred where the water supplies exceeded many times the recommended concentration of fluoride.

> **Other Causes of Mottled Enamel**
>
> *High fevers, or the use of certain antibiotics on very young children, may cause mottling of the permanent teeth. Why? The development of the tooth bud is temporarily interrupted, causing the permanent tooth to blemish.*

If your children have been drinking fluoridated water from birth, they could experience up to 65% less dental caries with no harmful effects.

The number of national and international organizations that support fluoridation are overwhelming, and include The American Dental Association, The American Heart Association, The American Medical Association, The United States Public Health Service, and The World Health Organization, and dozens more.* These organizations have investigated the case for fluoridation and they endorse it.

If the city in which you live has fluoride in your drinking water, you will probably observe that your children have a lower incidence of dental decay. If not, your children can still reap the benefits of fluoride. Ask your dentist if he can apply topical fluoride to your children's teeth or if they should be taking fluoride tablets. You can protect your children from decay and start them on practicing good preventive dentistry. And you can save yourself considerable money on dental bills, too.

Topical Fluoride Applications Will Prevent Your Children From Getting Any Decay.

"But Suzie got her fluorides, Doctor, why does she have a cavity?"

If your children have been drinking fluoridated water from birth, they could have up to two thirds less than the usual number of

---

*American Academy of Allergy, American Academy of Pediatrics, American Academy of Pedodontics, American Association for the Advancement of Science, American Association of Public Health Dentists, American Dental Hygienists Association, AFL-CIO, American Institute of Nutrition, American Legion, American Pharmaceutical Association, American Public Health Association, American School Health Association, American Society of Dentistry for Children, American Veterinary Medical Association, Canadian Dental Association, Canadian Medical Association, Canadian Public Health Association, Health Insurance Institute of America, International Dental Federation, National Congress of Parents & Teachers, National Health Council, National Research Council, Society of Toxology, U.S. Department of Defense.

dental caries. But even if your community doesn't have fluoridated water, you can still reduce the number of cavities by seeing that your children get *topical* applications of fluoride from their earliest dental visit, perhaps age two. That doesn't mean your child will NEVER get a cavity. Topical fluoride applications are effective in *reducing* cavities, but the amount of reduction varies from child to child. Topical fluorides do NOT constitute an innoculation against all decay in childhood. Of course, the earlier you start your child on these fluorides the better it is, because fluoride is only effective on a child's teeth *during the period of their eruption and growth*. Remember this: fluoride is effective only on developING teeth, not on developED teeth. That's why they are not given to adults whose teeth are already formed.

Some dentists believe that topical fluoride applications are valuable even if your child has been drinking fluoridated water all along. These topical fluorides are applied directly on your child's cleaned and dried teeth with a cotton swab, and there is no pain or discomfort to it. The applications should begin about age 2, and they should be repeated at the intervals your dentist recommends, usually about once a year until age 11 or 12. A single fluoride application may cost about $10 or a total of $100 over the entire ten year period. You can save many times that amount during your child's cavity prone years.

Fluoride toothpastes can help, too. If your child is taught to use them in conjunction with good tooth brushing habits, they can have a compounded value in reducing decay. You can start brushing your child's teeth using fluoride toothpaste as soon as he will accept the idea. Make a game of it so he will associate brushing with pleasure. Then he will get the idea and want to do the brushing himself.

Although there is not yet any known way to prevent all dental decay, a good diet, proper dental hygiene, and topical fluoride applications can reduce decay considerably. This means less cavities for your children and less money spent by you.

Gas is Better Than a Needle.

"Please, Doctor, put me to sleep. I don't want to feel anything." the retired businessman pleaded.

Many people who are especially fearful or anxious about their dental visit ask their dentist to "put them to sleep." They do this because they believe the common misconception that general anesthesia (being put to sleep) is superior to local anesthesia (commonly called novocaine, a shot, or a needle). These patients usually have an extremely low tolerance to any discomfort which they feel as pain, and they will do nearly anything to avoid it. While avoidance of pain is a human desire we all share, it is important to understand the differences between local and general anesthesia.

In *local* anesthesia, your dentist injects the anesthesia by needle into the gum to deaden or numb the area he will work on. The discomfort is brief and mild. You should then feel no pain and your dentist can even enter the nerve chamber of the tooth painlessly. Local anesthesia is by far safer, more efficient, and less costly than general anesthesia. It can be effective in almost every dental procedure, even in the setting of a broken jaw. Exceptions would occur where the dentist encounters totally uncooperative patients, the physically handicapped, the mentally disturbed, or those unable or unwilling to offer the dentist any cooperation. Local anesthesia is advantageous in that there is no "recovery period" needed to regain consciousness, and because you won't feel "woozy" or "dizzy" afterward. Also, there is no accompanying nausea or headache to follow. In fact, on leaving the dental chair, you can drive yourself home. Be careful not to bite your lips, cheeks or tongue while you are still numb. It could take several hours for the anesthesia to wear off.

General anesthesia is not as safe a procedure as local anesthesia. There is always that very small risk of anesthetic deaths, a statistical risk not to be ignored. The patient getting general anesthesia may be given a mask to inhale a gas until he is unconscious and "goes to sleep." Another form of general anesthesia is administered intravenously, usually by needle into the arm. Both methods require a deeper surgical plane and therefore a high degree of expertise, so they are not usually administered in the general dental office. They require special equipment and training. Therefore, patients who elect to have general anesthesia are referred to a specialist's office, or to a hospital where proper facilities and highly trained people are standing by. Obviously, this will be more expensive. Patients who have general anesthesia in the dental office may need to lie down for the "recovery period," and they may experience side effects, such as nausea and headache, after they have regained consciousness.

There is still another type of "gas,"* sometimes called laughing gas or analgesia, in which the patient is not totally asleep. This analgesia may be used in conjunction with a needle for particularly apprehensive patients. However, since it does not allow the patient to reach the high surgical plane of general anesthesia, it is safer.

> **No Laughing Matter**
>
> *In 1884, Dr. Horace Wells, an American dentist, demonstrated the properties of nitrous oxide or "laughing gas," by using it on himself while having his own tooth extracted.*

The newer machines for analgesia are now fully equipped with failsafe mechanisms which do not allow the patient to "go to sleep." Some general dental offices may have analgesia available, but again it will probably cost you more than the local anesthetic or shot.

As a general rule, it is to your advantage to choose the most conservative type of anesthetic, the simple local or "shot." It is safer and less expensive. Furthermore, it is easier for the dentist to work with local anesthetic because you are awake and can cooperate when your dentist asks you to rinse, turn your head, or open wider. Under general anesthesia where you are completely "out," you cannot offer any cooperation. Therefore, your mouth must be held open with mouth props and your throat must be packed with gauze to prevent any foreign body from being aspirated into your lungs. If you have the choice, pick local anesthesia.

To Relieve a Toothache, Rinse Your Mouth with Whiskey or Lay an Aspirin Beside the Tooth.

"I put an aspirin next to the tooth, but the pain didn't go away, Doctor," the railroad conductor said, holding one hand against his aching jaw.

*Nitrous oxide-oxygen analgesia.

These two home remedies to relieve a toothache are popular misconceptions that people have been trying for years. *They are NOT effective, are sometimes harmful, and often put off needed dental treatment, only aggravating the condition.*

Swishing whiskey around in your mouth and rinsing with it will do nothing to alleviate pain. Neither will an aspirin which is placed whole between the aching tooth and the cheek (not to be confused with swallowing an aspirin). As a matter of fact, the aspirin can cause considerable damage and increased pain. As it disintegrates slowly in your mouth, it may cause the delicate "gingival mucosa" or gum tissues to slough away, resulting in an ugly and painful sore dentists call "aspirin burn." It could take a week or ten days for that to heal, simply adding another painful complication to the distress of the toothache.

If you have pain, go to the dentist. Don't put it off hoping it will go away. Don't try to save money by making up your own home remedy or accepting the advice of a friend who guarantees success. That can only cause you more pain. And more money.

A Person is Born to Have Good Teeth or Bad Teeth and There's Nothing You Can do About it.

"My mother's side of the family all have bad teeth, so there's nothing much I can do about it," the young copywriter told me. "I guess I just inherited my troubles from them."

Many people blame all their dental troubles on their parents who "gave" them bad teeth. This is a misconception that people accept when they feel the condition of their mouth is hopeless and nothing can be done for them. There are definite measures you can take to prevent dental disease and there are effective ways to combat those dental problems that are unavoidable.

Of course we do inherit certain characteristics from our parents. It's not uncommon to see a child whose facial characteristics resemble his mother or father. "She's a dead ringer for her father," (or grandfather or aunt) is a common expression of this family resemblance. The size and shape of the jaw bone, and the position of the teeth in the arch, may be the result of your genes, and there appears to be a tendency for "supernumerary" (extra) teeth or congenitally missing teeth to run in a family. *But "bad" or "good" teeth are not settled by the fates. They are the result of many factors and variables over which YOU have control.*

Your dental health is largely your own responsibility. Although dental diseases cannot be eliminated, you can do a lot to assure your own natural teeth's good health through proper diet, and scrupulous hygiene. Even if your parents had terrible teeth, you can reduce the odds and strike out against decay. It's certainly wiser and less costly to prevent dental disease than to pay for the repairs after the damage is there. You can maintain good health and extend the life of your own teeth through regular dental checkups. *No one is doomed because their parents had bad teeth.*

● ● ● ● ●

There is one final myth we must deal with that persists despite the lack of ANY scientific evidence whatsoever to support it. I have searched the literature, and conferred with patients, specialists, and professors in dental schools. Clearly there is absolutely not a shred of evidence, nor data, nor laboratory tests to even suggest its authority. In a quarter century of clinical practice of dentistry, I must have heard it hundreds and hundreds of times. My colleagues, too, report it from their private offices, hospitals, and community clinics. It appears to be rampant among my younger patients — those in the age three to eight category — and both boys and girls are equally convinced of its absolute authority and dependability.

If You Leave Your Tooth Under Your Pillow, When You Wake up The Tooth Fairy Will Replace it With a Quarter.

Having seen the quarters clutched in small hands, and having heard the trusting and sincere reports of my younger patients, I am convinced *this is one myth that is absolutely true!*

THERE IS A TOOTH FAIRY.

5
Check Your Dentist's Fees Against the Averages

One out of two Americans is likely to duck a checkup with his dentist out of fear of pain or a tremendous bill. If you've avoided your dentist, trying to stave off another bombardment to your budget, you have lots of company. Most people fear dental bills because they know nothing about the fees they might be charged. The same consumers who can rattle off the prices of a can of peas, a local movie ticket, or a gallon of gasoline, are lost when it comes to the cost of a dental service. Once they open wide, they fear they have also opened their wallets, their checking accounts, and even their piggy banks.

If you've put off seeing your dentist because you don't know what's in store for you financially, there are lots of facts you can tuck away in your head to lessen that uncertainty. Although fees vary from dentist to dentist, from city to city, and from large urban areas (higher) to small rural areas (lower), you can become acquainted with *the range of fees for the most common procedures* so that you have some idea of what to expect. You don't have to memorize the fee for a subperiosteal implant — that's rare, so chances are you won't have one. But it helps to know what the average fee is for a filling, an upper denture, or a crown. If you have a clearer picture, you're at an advantage.

Understand, for example, that *the fee for a filling* is NOT the same as *the fee for filling a tooth*. It's easy to misunderstand, to assume (incorrectly) that if you need five fillings, five teeth will be treated. A filling generally means a *surface* of a tooth. There are five surfaces to a tooth: the biting side ("occlusal"); the side toward the midline ("mesial"); the side away from the midline ("distal"); the side toward the face ("facial"); and the side toward the tongue ("lingual"). Therefore, if your dentist bills you for five fillings, he worked on *five surfaces,* but perhaps on only two or three teeth. Just as a waitress calls out, "BLT, hold the mayo" (bacon, lettuce, and tomato without mayonnaise), your dentist may say, "an MOD" (mesial, occlusal, distal). That means *three surfaces to be filled on one tooth.* You will be charged for *three fillings.*

Consumerism Produces Fee Surveys

In 1973, the American Dental Association Bureau of Economic Research and Statistics published a survey of *Dental Fees for General Practitioners (not* specialists) *in the United States.* It covered 139 dental services, many you probably never heard of, and listed the mean (average) fee for each one. It also noted the number of dentists who answered *each* question and the standard deviation (range) in dollars and cents for each fee.

For example, in Question 124, the service was described as "Incision and drainage of abscess, intraoral." 861 dentists responded to that question and the average fee was $13.66, with a range from $5 to $25. Does that help the consumer? Probably not much. To the average dental consumer, the five page report appears to be a muddle of incomprehensible data. The report itself carries the warning that some of the statistics should be used with caution. Why?

In 1973, there were about 110,000 dentists practicing in the United States. The fees established for Question 124, for example, were based on answers from only 861 dentists. You don't need a computer analyst to realize what a small sample that is. Even a fee established for a question answered by as many as 2646 dentists (the highest figure in the survey) represents only about 2% of the dentists in this country. How accurately, then, does the survey reflect what you as a consumer can expect to pay? Suppose the other 98% of dentists had answered, how would those average fees have changed?

In addition to the problems of a small sample, this *American Dental Association Survey* reflects fees established in 1973. It is not adjusted for skyrocketing increases in the cost of living. Also, the fees range widely depending upon which of the fifty states you live in. If you lived in Alaska in 1973, a cleaning might have cost you $20. In Alabama, $9. A porcelain crown might have cost $143 in New Jersey. In Idaho, $84. What's a poor consumer to do?

First, become familiar with dental terminology, procedures, and treatments through self-education. Next, ask your dentist what his fee is before proceeding with your work. Don't accept an all-inclusive fee that merely states: "For Professional Services . . . $115." Ask for a breakdown on how that $115 was arrived at. *Ask! Don't be in awe of your dentist.*

Become consumer oriented. Although the *American Dental Association Fee Survey* may be too dentist-oriented for you to understand, a number of nonprofessional magazines have printed "boiled down versions" that cover the fees for the most common procedures. Both *Reader's Digest* and *Consumer Reports* did this for their readers. Many of the mass circulation magazines like *Esquire* and *Glamour* have published articles dealing with dental consumerism — what dental services will cost you, comparisons of dental fees, and how to get more for your money.

Be alert to newspapers, too. Their articles are slanted toward the average consumer and are written in readable lay terminology. From *The New York Times* to *The San Juan Star,* articles on medical-dental subjects have been appearing frequently, and many newspapers are adding columns like *The Newark Star Ledger's* "Health and Medicine" to educate their readers. Perhaps your local newspaper carries such a column. Watch for the television programs that feature consumer reports added to their news coverage. Follow the TV specials and documentaries on health subjects. They can fill in a lot of information for you.

Look over the different surveys on dental fees. Although there's more to reading a chart than simply memorizing fees, you can check your own dentist's fees against the averages. Here is an updated, "boiled down version" of the *American Dental Association's 1975 Fee Survey* averaged for all 50 states. It is the most recent available and covers the most common treatments. Keep in mind:

1. These are average fees. They're probably higher in urban than rural areas.

2. Fees are NOT adjusted for an inflation factor since 1975.
3. This covers 15 treatments (rounded to the nearest dollar) by general practitioners *not* specialists.

AVERAGE FEES FOR 15 COMMON DENTAL PROCEDURES

Based on the 1975 *American Dental Association* Fee Schedule of *general* dentists in all 50 states. Remember these figures rounded to the nearest dollar represent 1975 fees, and you should adjust them for a realistic inflation factor.

Common Dental Procedure	Low Fee	High Fee	National Average
Initial exam	0	17	8
Complete X ray series	16	30	22
Cleaning (prophylaxis)	10	20	14
Silver filling (one surface)	7	15	10
Silver filling (two surfaces)	10	20	15
Gold Inlay (two surfaces)	60	150	96*
Gingivectomy (gum surgery per quadrant)	30	150	70
Porcelain crown (with metal)	140	250	179*
Root canal therapy (one canal)	70	125	92
Root canal therapy (two canals)	90	165	120
Full upper denture	175	350	251
Removable partial denture with two clasps	150	375	242
Fixed bridge (replacing one tooth; 3 units porcelain fused to gold)	400	750	535*
Simple extraction	10	20	13
Extraction of impacted wisdom tooth	40	100	64

*These items use gold, and world gold prices fluctuate.

No survey evaluates the *quality* of the work performed, so the price range can be considerably wide. However, to simply choose a dentist based on the lowest fee is to discount the quality of the treatment. That can be dangerous.

Most important, don't abdicate your responsibility. *Be your own consumer advocate.* Consumer groups are springing up all over the country. You may wish to join one. Many of these groups are compiling directories of useful information for the benefit of consumers. They list the names of dentists and information on their fees and services.

The Health Research Group, a unit of Ralph Nader's Public Citizen, Inc., came out with a directory of Washington, D.C. dentists in 1974. Both *The Wall Street Journal* and *The Washington Post* applauded the directory as one step toward eliminating artificially high professional fees. Here are some of the fees uncovered by the probe of Nader's Raiders.

\multicolumn{3}{c}{**NADER'S SURVEY OF WASHINGTON D.C. DENTISTS – 1974**}		
Service	Average	Range
Initial exam	$28	$10-75
Full mouth survey	$23	$15-35
Prophylaxis (cleaning)	$16	$0-25
Silver filling (2 surfaces)	$18	$8-30
Upper *and* lower dentures	$545	$400-1000
Root Canal (anteriors)	$87	$65-125
Plaque control	$24	$0-85
Add inflation factor to 1974 fees.		

Like most surveys, this one has holes in it, too. Undertaken in August-September, 1974, it yielded only 44 dentists who would give their fees — only about 10% of the 430 dentists contacted. (The American Dental Association listed 690 dentists in Washington, D.C.) This raises the question of how much a published fee actually reveals to the patient. It's a complicated business because some of the fees don't take into account who is doing the service (a hygienist may be giving the cleaning), how difficult the same service may be for different patients, or the additional services included under one procedure.

Examination fees have been listed from $10 to $75. Complete dentures from $400 to $1000. It's not easy for you, the consumer, to measure the quality of dental care and it would be dangerous to conclude that the best dentistry is the cheapest. That could prove a costly and painful mistake. According to the 1975 *American Dental Association Survey,* a patient could expect to pay about $251 for a denture. But Mrs. H. P. of Frackville, Pennsylvania reports she paid only $40 at the Sexton-Shealy Clinic in Florence, South Carolina. Did she get a bargain?

In spite of their shortcomings, surveys by consumer groups can serve you because *they encourage dentist's accountability.* Consumers who feel dentists don't police themselves properly are not alone. Dr. David R. Bishop, a Washington, D.C. dentist, agrees. "There should be more policing," he insists. "If I were a patient, I would like to know, for example, if a dentist used a lead apron. I know many dentists who don't or who take other shortcuts in their practices. The American Dental Association is too politically oriented to take steps to correct this." It is interesting to note that the *American Dental Association Survey* indicated that nearly half of all dentists never take the lead bib precaution. You may well wonder what's done about it? Does the dentist receive a fine or reprimand? The answer is no.

Another dentist, Dr. David H. Frome of Silver Springs, Maryland, who served as a consultant to the *Washington, D.C. Survey* says, "If the dental profession can not or will not undertake the project of educating the public on how to select a dentist, then consumer organizations will fill the need."

Objections to surveys abound. Some say the most obvious flaw in any survey is that it has to be updated constantly or it grows stale. Many critics feel surveys are only a symptom of the overall wariness of today's consumers and serve no purpose. Others admit the surveys do have some useful features because they are progressive, and they deserve a place in the consumer movement.

The Washington, D.C. directory titled "Taking The Pain Out of Finding A Good Dentist" has set off firecrackers. Over 30 cities have planned similar directories using the Washington, D.C. survey as a model. Pittsburgh, New York, Nashville, Louisville, Philadelphia, Los Angeles, Milwaukee, Denver, Atlanta, San Juan, Chicago,

San Francisco, Jersey City, Dallas, Boston, Cleveland, and Omaha have all jumped on the bandwagon.

In 1974, the state of Connecticut issued its own "Consumer's Guide to Dentistry." It was printed as a public service by AETNA Life and Casualty Insurance Company. The Connecticut Citizens Action Group and The Connecticut Research Group were two citizen groups that joined the Connecticut State Dental Association to produce the 16 page guide of useful consumer information. Anyone interested in the table of fees for Connecticut dentists may write to:

The Connecticut Citizen Action Group
P.O. Box 6465
Hartford, Conn. 06106

Perhaps your city or state has such a guide or is planning one.

How Your Bill is Determined

Patients often wonder *what goes into their bills.* How does your dentist establish the fee for a particular procedure? Why do fees vary so widely from office to office? Like any other businessman in a free enterprise system, your dentist establishes fees according to the competition of the marketplace and his desire for a realistic return on his investment. What has he invested? After high school, he has probably spent six to eight years in higher education, first in college, then in a graduate school of dentistry before he is awarded his D.D.S. (or D.M.D.). This has cost him thousands of dollars in educational expenses *plus* the loss of income he might have been earning over that six to eight year period. Add to this the expense of setting up his practice — special dental chairs, cabinets, instruments, X rays, furniture, and supplies — and it's not unrealistic to conclude that he has invested well over $100,000 before he's ready to charge for his first filling.

Obviously, like any other businessman, he wants to recoup his initial capital investment. A portion of this is reflected in your bill. Other expenses included in the average fee are laboratory fees which could represent one fourth of your bill. The crown for which you paid $200 may have cost him $50 to pay his laboratory technician for fabricating the crown. Add to that the rent, utilities, billing costs, employee salaries, and dental supplies, too. These all go into determining your bill. Obviously, inflation raises his costs too, and this is also reflected back to you. So be careful in checking a survey to add 10-15% because there is a time lag of two years between gathering and documenting those fees before they get to you.

Many progressive dentists try to keep up with the newest developments in their field by taking advanced courses in special techniques. Continuing education courses cost them money as well as loss of income if they must be out of their office for days or weeks. They must also replace outmoded equipment for newer equipment and keep abreast of finer diagnostic models as they come out. If your dentist uses a special Panorex Scanner X ray in addition to the traditional X ray, he may have spent $12,000 for that single item.

Considering all this does not, however, make it any easier for you when it comes time to pay your bills. What *will* make it easier? How can you avoid overcharges? How can you deal with frauds and incompetents?

> **Governor Finds 15% of Dentists to be Frauds**
>
> *The Pennsylvania Insurance Department booklet endorsed by Governor Milton J. Shapp states: "Based on available evidence, it can be conservatively estimated that at least 15% (of U.S. dentists) are incompetent, dishonest, or both."*

What alternatives are there if you can't afford the fee a private dentist has quoted you?

If your dentist has quoted a fee, and you can't see your way clear to laying out that much money, first talk it over with him. Ask him to reconsider the procedure he has suggested for a less expensive one that may serve your purpose just as well. A simple amalgam filling could cost about $10, a gold filling $80. Do you really need gold when amalgam might do as well? If you've had four teeth extracted and your dentist suggests a *fixed* bridge replacement at a cost of $1200, ask him if there is a less expensive way of doing it. A *removable* bridge at $225 might serve as well. Savings? $975. If you're still unhappy, seek another opinion.

You may even decide to change dentists. 15 out of every 100 patients switch to another practitioner. A New York City high school student switched because his dentist "strung out the work." A Des Moines, Iowa mother switched because she received a bill for $40 after she was told the work would be $20. "I had the dentist budgeted for $20," she complained. A Newark, New Jersey lawyer switched when he received a bill for $200 after being told the work would cost $100. "The man simply said the work cost more than he anticipated. If I went around giving those kinds of reasons," he moaned, "I'd never get a client."

If you have a dispute over a fee, talk it over with your dentist and ask him to make an adjustment. Even if you've agreed on the amount of the fee, there may be a misunderstanding over the *way* you plan to pay it. "I was two weeks late with my payment and this guy was on my back," was the reason one patient switched. If you feel you've been wronged, tell your dentist. It could be a simple mistake in billing.

Group Practices

Most dentists — about 4 out of 5 — are in solo practice (they work alone or with a dental assistant). However, a growing phenomenon has sprung up in recent years called the "group practice." That can mean something to you. Dentists in a group practice who work together under one roof, sharing facilities and personnel, may give you certain advantages. Although their fees may not be lower, *you may be getting more for your money*. Dentists in a group practice are more likely to keep the quality of their work high because their colleagues are looking over their shoulder. There is accountability and on the spot peer review. Callousness or incompetency would not likely be tolerated.

The exceptions to watch out for are the "dental sweatshops" or "extraction mills," where groups of dentists practice together unscrupulously, usually in low income urban areas where they can foist unnecessary cheap work on their uninformed patients. Some Medicaid type groups seem to have one avowed purpose in mind: to feather their own nests by getting the greatest number of patients in and out as fast as possible. You can imagine the quality of the work performed there.

However, in a competent group practice, often located in upper-income suburbs, dentists practice together, delivering first class dentistry. You can get many advantages from such groups. These dentists "cover" for each other in emergencies, on weekends, or when one is away on vacation. They also keep a total record of your full dental picture on hand, and if they are in different specialties, you have "one-stop-shopping." A single office can give your toddler his fluorides (the pedodontist), straighten your teenager's teeth (the orthodontist), and treat your own gums (the periodontist). In a well run group practice you can benefit from the range and depth of the accumulated experience of the entire group, and each dentist can confer with the other at a moment's notice. Since two or three dentists share expenses, they are likely to purchase the most sophisticated equipment and diagnostic tools that would be prohibitive to the dentist in solo practice.

On the other hand, even the best group practices may become so large that you feel "depersonalized." Watch out for the ultra-efficient, high powered group practices which approach the atmosphere of a mini-hospital. Those dentists may lose the human touch. To them you are a chart number, and they may not even know your name.

The Dental School Clinic

What other alternatives are there? If you can't afford a private dentist, where can you go? You don't have dental insurance through your employer and you can't afford to pay. Maybe you have a limited income, a small pension, or social security which doesn't go far in today's marketplace. What's left?

Dental schools are scattered throughout the country. They operate clinics, usually in large cities like New York, Boston, or Philadelphia. If you live near a dental school, consider having your work done by a student dentist who is overseen by his professors who check off each step of the procedure. Naturally, that can take a long time and seem to stretch to eternity. You may have to come back half a dozen times for a procedure that a private dentist would complete in one visit. *But you can save money.*

At the first visit the student dentist may only take your history. The second visit may be for X rays. The third visit may be a clinical examination of your mouth. On the fourth visit you might be advised of the treatment plan, the number of your appointments, and the fees. So it is possible that you will not actually be worked on until the fifth visit. If you are traveling on two buses each way, the time and carfare can add up. But if you're short on money and have an abundance of time (and patience), you can get your work done at a relatively low cost. Some consumer articles suggest that since professors are looking over their students' work, you are *bound* to get superior dentistry. That doesn't necessarily follow. But if money is a problem, you might find that the dental school clinic can save you hundreds of dollars.

For example, a New Jersey Dental School Clinic charges only $15 for the following services: a full series X ray (18 views); a Panorex X ray; an admission and medical history; a clinical examination of your mouth by a student dentist and a professor; a written estimate of the fees; and a treatment plan with the number of appointments noted. This might easily amount to $40 in a private office. However, the clinic might also stretch out these services over four or five visits. So if you *can't* afford the money, but you *can* afford the time, a dental school clinic might be for you. A one surface filling might cost only $4 (up to $15 in a private office); root canals, $25 (up to $250 in a private office); and a full upper or lower denture, only $50 including two adjustments (up to $500 in a private office). And if your case presents a unique educational experience to a student (who has perhaps studied your type of case in a textbook), the dental school clinic may waive the entire fee.

IS THERE A DENTAL SCHOOL NEAR YOU?

School of Dentistry,
University of Alabama
1919 Seventh Avenue, South
Birmingham 35233

School of Dentistry
University of the Pacific
2155 Webster Street
San Francisco 94115

School of Dentistry
University of California
San Francisco Medical Center
San Francisco 94103

School of Dentistry
University of California
at Los Angeles
Medical Center
Los Angeles 90024

School of Dentistry
University of Southern California
925 West Thirty-Fourth Street
Los Angeles 90007

School of Dentistry
Loma Linda University
Loma Linda 92354

School of Dentistry
University of Colorado
Medical Center
4200 East Ninth Avenue
Denver 80220

University of Connecticut
 Health Center
School of Dental Medicine
263 Farmington Avenue
Farmington 06032

School of Dentistry
Georgetown University
3900 Reservoir Road, N.W.
Washington 20007

College of Dentistry
Howard University
600 W Street, N.W.
Washington 20001

College of Dentistry
J. Hillis Miller Health Center
University of Florida
Gainesville 32603

School of Dentistry
Emory University
106 Forrest Avenue, N.E.
Atlanta 30329

School of Dentistry
Medical College of Georgia
Augusta 30904

School of Dentistry
Loyola University of Chicago
1757 West Harrison Street
Chicago 60612

Northwestern University Dental School
311 East Chicago Avenue
Chicago 60611

College of Dentistry
University of Illinois
808 South Wood Street
Chicago 60612

Southern Illinois University
School of Dentistry
Edwardsville 62025

School of Dentistry
Indiana University
1121 West Michigan Street
Indianapolis 46202

College of Dentistry
The University of Iowa
Dental Building
Iowa City 52240

College of Dentistry
University of Kentucky
Medical Center
Lexington 40506

School of Dentistry
University of Louisville
129 East Broadway
Louisville 40202

School of Dentistry
Loyola University of New Orleans
6363 Saint Charles Avenue
New Orleans 70118

School of Dentistry
Louisiana State University
Medical Center
1190 Florida Avenue, Building 101
New Orleans 70019

School of Dentistry
University of Maryland
666 West Baltimore Street
Baltimore 21201

Harvard School of Dental Medicine
188 Longwood Avenue
Boston 02115

Tufts University
School of Dental Medicine
136 Harrison Avenue
Boston 02111

Boston University
School of Graduate Dentistry
100 East Newton Street
Boston 02118

University of Michigan
School of Dentistry
Ann Arbor 48104

University of Detroit
School of Dentistry
2985 East Jefferson Avenue
Detroit 48207

University of Mississippi Medical Center
School of Dentistry
2500 North State Street
Jackson 39216

University of Minnesota
Washington Avenue & Union Street, S.E.
Minneapolis 55455

School of Dentistry
University of Missouri at Kansas City
1108 East Tenth Street
Kansas City 64106

School of Dentistry
St. Louis University
3556 Caroline Street
St. Louis 63104

School of Dentistry
Washington University
4559 Scott Avenue
St. Louis 63110

Boyne School of Dental Science
Creighton University
26th & California Streets
Omaha 68131

College of Dentistry
University of Nebraska
40th & Holdrege Streets
Lincoln 68503

New Jersey College of Medicine
 and Dentistry
100 Bergen Street
Newark 07101

School of Dentistry
Fairleigh Dickinson University
Teaneck, New Jersey 07666

School of Dental and Oral Surgery
Columbia University
630 West 168th Street
New York 10032

College of Dentistry
New York University
421 First Avenue
New York 10010

College of Dentistry
State University of New York
 at Buffalo
Capen Hall, 15 The Circle
Buffalo 14214

School of Dentistry
State University of New York
 at Stony Brook
Health Sciences Center
Stony Brook 11790

School of Dentistry
University of North Carolina
Post Office Box 750
Chapel Hill 27514

74 HOW TO SAVE YOUR TEETH AND YOUR MONEY

College of Dentistry
The Ohio State University
305 West Twelfth Avenue
Columbus 43210

School of Dentistry
Case Western Reserve University
2165 Adelbert Road
Cleveland 44106

University of Oklahoma
College of Dentistry
Health Science Center
P.O. Box 26901
Oklahoma City 73190

University of Oregon Dental School
6111 S.W. Campus Drive
Sam Jack Park
Portland 97201

School of Dentistry
Temple University
3223 North Broad Street
Philadelphia 19140

School of Dental Medicine
University of Pennsylvania
4001 Spruce Street
Philadelphia 19104

School of Dental Medicine
University of Pittsburgh
Thackeray and O'Hara Streets
Pittsburgh 15213

School of Dentistry
University of Puerto Rico
San Juan 00905

Medical University of South Carolina
80 Barre Street
Charleston 29401

School of Dentistry
Meharry Medical College
1005 Eighteenth Avenue, North
Nashville 37208

College of Dentistry
University of Tennessee
62 South Dunlap Street
Memphis 38103

College of Dentistry
Baylor University
800 Hall Street
Dallas 75226

The University of Texas Dental Ranch
6516 John Freeman Avenue
Houston 77025

University of Texas Dental School
7703 Floyd Curl Drive
San Antonio 78229

School of Dentistry
Virginia Commonwealth University
Wood Memorial Building
521 North Eleventh Street
Richmond 23219

School of Dentistry
University of Washington
Health Sciences Building
Seattle 98105

School of Dentistry
West Virginia University
The Medical Center
Morgantown 26506

School of Dentistry
Marquette University
604 North Sixteenth Street
Milwaukee 53233

Government Clinics

In 1974, 95% of the people who sought dental treatment went to one of 110,000 private dentists in this country. Over 80% of the population lives in an area where there is one dentist for every 3,000 people. So most Americans — four out of five — have a private dentist available to them. *If they can afford it.* And there's the rub! Suppose they can't? Where can the great numbers of needy people go to get dental care? That's where the free government clinics come in.

Many state and local governments offer health department clinics that supply dental services to the poor at very reduced costs or even free. Programs like Head Start and Medicaid have established neighborhood dental clinics in housing developments and hospitals to perform free dentistry for the indigent and handicapped. Welfare offices and voluntary organizations also sponsor free clinics. How effective are they? What is the quality of their work? How many do they serve?

The rationale for establishing a free clinic is generally to locate the facility in an area with a high concentration of poor people who need care, but can't afford it. So government funds (your taxes) will provide the facility, and the needy can get the care free (or almost free). It seems simple and logical. On paper it would appear that everyone eligible would flock to it. But reports show that quite the opposite can occur. In St. Paul-Minneapolis, the free clinic averaged only 23% utilization. This clinic was in the heart of a depressed area where private dental care was out of the question. A clinic located in Roxbury, Massachusetts experienced an even lower usage. A Hoboken, New Jersey clinic closed its doors because so few people used it. Why?

Often these clinics are not managed responsibly. This produces an intense antagonism between the dentists and their patients. Patients complain that when they come to the clinic, their appointments have been cancelled or rescheduled. They are frustrated by dentists who practice "pacing" or "goldbricking" — holding down the number of appointments to a minimum. Their work drags on endlessly with a series of temporary fillings and a different dentist assigned at every appointment. There is no dentist-patient relationship established, and they are kept waiting for hours.

Dentists complain that the patients have no sense of responsibility toward meeting their appointments. They don't show up, forget, or don't care. They don't follow instructions in their treatment, are uncooperative, even hostile. Some of these dentists claim they fear for their own safety. Result? They "give up," convinced that little can be done. A Newark, New Jersey dentist associated with a municipal dental clinic for many years finally quit, saying, "What's the sense of filling their teeth? They come into the clinic chewing a candy bar and they don't even own a toothbrush. It's like spitting in the ocean to raise the tide."

> **A Losing Battle**
>
> *It has been estimated that approximately 80% of the children from the lowest socioeconomic class have no toothbrush of their own.*

In such an atmosphere, it is not surprising that some of these clinics fold up.

Even under the best conditions, government sponsored clinics leave something to be desired. Most cover urgent, pressing services, like filling and extracting painful teeth. But more sophisticated procedures like periodontal treatments or orthodontic treatments are scarce. People who need emergency care wait in pain for days or longer. If the clinic closes at 4:30 on Friday and a patient develops a toothache at 5:00, he must wait until Monday (if he's lucky) for relief. The indignity of dirty waiting rooms, hard benches, and indifference among some of the personnel — dentists, assistants, and petty bureaucrats — does *not* bring out the best in dental care. Some clinics are adequate, but rarely do the poor get what the private patient gets. So while a fee to a private dentist doesn't guarantee first class dentistry, it appears that a free clinic and the absence of a fee rarely bring out the best.

There is one other phenomenon that the poor resort to in order to get cheap dentistry: Denturism (using an unlicensed "dental mechanic" to make cheap dentures). This is illegal in every state.* The laboratory technician or "dental mechanic" is licensed *only* to fabricate a denture according to the dentist's prescription. He is operating illegally if he takes impressions in the mouth and fits dentures.

*Dental mechanics in some states are lobbying hard to change this.

Private Interest Clinics

How can the vast number of working people wrestling with tight budgets get lower cost quality dentistry? One answer has come from *private interest clinics,* such as unions or employee groups. They have organized their own private dental clinics as additional benefits to their members. In some cases, the coverage may also extend to the member's spouse and family. These private interest clinics have stepped in hoping to lower the costs of private dental care for their members who will no longer go to a private dentist and pay his fee. How does it work?

The union or group may set up their own clinic, buy their own equipment, and hire their own salaried dentists and personnel strictly for the use of their members. The rationale here is to cut the costs of delivering dental care through shared expenses and controlled conditions. Does it work? Sometimes yes, sometimes no. In some states, clinic operators did not deliver what they promised, and legal loopholes allowed them to get away with it. Unfortunately, these privately established clinics suffered from many of the same pains as government sponsored clinics including "pacing" and rampant bureaucratic red tape. Dentists on salary are not likely to produce maximum work. Whether they see five patients or twenty-five a day, they earn the same salary. A few nasty cases resulted in broken contracts and refusal to pay premiums.

Some unions now prefer a plan where their members pick their own private dentist and the union pays up to 90% of the fee.* On the other hand, despite these problems, there are also some responsibly run clinics to point to. A successful Los Angeles clinic, for example, operates two such facilities, and each one treats about 500 patients per day. Utilization is high — about 70% of those eligible come in to be treated by the 36 dentists and 4 specialists. The waiting period is four to six weeks. It appears to be working well.

Cut-Rate Dentistry

Suppose you aren't rich, you aren't eligible for a free clinic, and you don't belong to a union (or employer) dental plan. There is still

*See Chapter 7 on dental insurance.

one more choice open to you: the low cost-high volume "assembly line" dental practice.

These offices basically supply "take-em-out, put-em-in" dental services where mass produced techniques keep the costs down. You won't be able to get sophisticated dentistry such as orthodontia, periodontia, or endodontia, but if you need a denture (and extractions) you could probably get one for about $50, whereas a private dentist might charge $500. These high volume groups deliver low overhead bargain dentistry, and specialize in super fast extractions and cheap dentures. A man in his mid-thirties reported his experiences at such an "extraction mill." All his teeth were extracted in about 35 seconds and the dentist said, "This is just like shelling corn." Such offices are big business. The annual gross earnings for one of the most successful ones was reported to be around the 4 million dollar mark.*

Patients start lining up for their while-you-wait dentures at 3:00 A.M. the night before, and they may come from hundreds of miles away. Why? They flock to these "dental factories" to get cheap dentistry in the belief that their new *cut-rate denture* is a great bargain. They think they have gotten rid of all future dental problems for $50 — because their natural teeth were extracted. They believe that a full denture is the answer to all their problems, a passport to a trouble-free mouth.

The big unanswered question is: "Did those teeth that were extracted *like shelling corn* really have to come out?" In many cases, the patient himself makes the diagnosis when he says, "Take them all out, Doc, I want false teeth." Even if the *cut-rate denture* is comfortable, such unnecessary mass extractions are no bargain in dental health. On the other hand, for edentulous (without any teeth) patients who *don't* need extractions and *don't* have $500 to spend, a low cost, acceptable denture is better than nothing. If you can afford a $20 filet mignon at a plush restaurant, you can buy first class dining. But if you can only afford a hamburger and a milkshake at McDonalds, it beats going hungry.

In order to get first hand information directly from an "extraction mill," we wrote to the Sexton Dental Clinic of Florence, South

---

*The Sexton-Shealy Clinic.

Carolina and asked for information about having "teeth pulled" and "the cost for uppers and lowers." They answered:

> "Upper and lower dentures are $50. An upper or lower denture alone is $30. Extractions are $3 each, medication is between $3 and $6. We make a plastic partial for $40. We also make a cast metal partial which requires 2 trips to the clinic about 3 weeks apart and the cost of this is between $135 and $150. No personal checks please."

Their letter (signed H. L. Eagerton, Jr. D.D.S.) advised us to arrive "at 3:00 am in the morning" and that "There are two motels connected with the clinic." Stamped at the bottom of the letter was this:

> "CITY ORDINANCES PROHIBIT OVERNIGHT PARKING OF TRAILERS OR CAMPERS IN THE PARKING LOT."

That's cut rate dentistry!

HMOs: Another Alternative

HMO stands for Health Maintenance Organization, and it is basically a prepaid health plan that permits a family to pay *one fixed price* for all its health services rather than pay for each visit. It's not a new concept. Among the early Chinese dynasties, the doctor's livelihood depended upon his keeping his patients in good health, so as long as they were healthy he prospered. Most HMOs grew rapidly in the 1970's, in response to consumer and labor union demands. Today there are hundreds of plans which serve about 5% of the population, despite the opposition of organized medicine. The American Medical Association has opposed the expansion of the plans because they require doctors to work for a fixed salary instead of a fee-for-service arrangement. But with new rules requiring employers with more than 25 workers to offer plans,* it looks like they will continue to expand.

In 1971, there were less than 30 HMO groups, representing only 1% of the dentists in the United States. Most HMOs continue to be

*If a government-approved plan is available in the area.

medical practices. Some date back to the twenties, but few offer dentistry as a supplement.

The dental HMO is a relatively new concept in which a group of dentists get together, as in a group practice. But instead of charging for each visit, the patient pays one overall fee that covers their work *regardless of the number of visits.* The dental HMO is in its infancy, but there appears to be a trend in this direction. Most arose out of the need to deal with the spiraling expenses of dental health which take a larger and larger chunk out of your consumer dollars. What are the benefits to you?

A study by Dr. Max Schoen has shown that a prepayment plan has additional benefits besides reducing the costs of your dental budget. HMOs reported a reduced number of dental extractions over the traditional fee-for-service arrangement. Dentists who combine their resources into HMO groups can also offer certain increased services, such as better preventive care. And patients who might hesitate to spend money on preventive dentistry, because they have to pay for each visit, might be more likely to see the dentist *more often and preventively* in an HMO since their overall fee covers everything. Although it's not a perfect way to dispense dental health care, it offers certain benefits according to Dr. Fred Troxel, an HMO dentist who lives in a farmhouse 20 miles outside of Rochester, New York. He thinks HMOs are better for the consumer.

"Many of our patients have not been to the dentist in the past except for extractions. Here we provide comprehensive health care for them and take time to show them how they can avoid losing another tooth." He adds, too, "Our fees are very reasonable."

You may wonder what kind of dentist would forgo a fee-for-service practice to work as a salaried employee in an HMO? Dr. Troxel says a community sensitive dentist would find an HMO attractive. "It's not for those looking for an easy buck either. Extra work will not increase your earnings."

Since the dental HMO is basically a new concept, it will probably go through its share of growing pains. But Dr. Troxel says: "We are in the community and therefore more available. We put every patient through a preventive program before actual treatment begins, except, of course, in an emergency. We also have a recall system and further enforcement of patient education programs to insure dental care isn't a one-shot affair." You may wish to investigate the advantages of an HMO for your family.

Quality Control: Are You Getting What You Paid For?

It's difficult for a dental consumer to check on the quality of work he receives, so most dental care is built on trust. But that shouldn't mean *blind* trust.

Early in 1976, a series of five *New York Times* articles revealed that 16,000 doctors (or 5% of the 320,000 in the United States) were *unfit to practice.* Findings indicate that 2.4 million unnecessary operations are performed each year in which nearly 12,000 patients die; 10,000 patients die or suffer from antibiotic reactions to doctors' prescriptions; 260,000 women undergo needless hysterectomies each year; and half a million children undergo unwarranted surgery. Because medicine has been largely steeped in myth and is closed to public investigation, only 66 doctors, on the average, lose their licenses each year.* Given this overwhelming evidence of misjudgment, greed, drug addiction, alcoholism, mismanagement, and incompetence among physicians, are you willing to believe that dentists are any better? If, like physicians, only 5% of dentists are unfit, then there are perhaps 6,000 unfit dentists practicing in the United States. Obviously, life and death decisions are not nearly as likely among dentists as among physicians. Still, wouldn't you like to protect yourself against dental incompetence? Can you afford to turn yourself over *in blind faith?*

Although you can't judge your dentist's technical skills or know whether his diagnosis was correct or his treatment appropriate, there are certain things you can check on. There are ways you can distinguish bad dentistry from good dentistry and tell if you're being "oversold."

A good dentist will have a light touch and make every effort to reduce your discomfort during injections by applying a topical anesthetic first. If prolonged drilling is required, he'll pause for you to rest your jaw joint and relax. During drilling, he'll cool the drill with a water spray to reduce the heat. In filling a tooth or placing a crown, he will attempt to keep the area being worked on free of saliva. Most dentists use cotton rolls for this or a saliva ejector

*0.02 of 1%.

which sucks the saliva out. Others (less frequently) use a rubber dam, a rectangular piece of rubber used to isolate the tooth from the rest of the mouth.

Once a restoration is completed, a good dentist will polish a filling to make it look better and feel smoother. He will contour the filling so it feels comfortable and is not too high. Fillings should not fall out or crack easily. Porcelain and composite resins (white fillings) should last four to five years; amalgam (silver fillings) can last longer.* Crowns and fixed bridges, assuming you're practicing good oral hygiene, can last ten years or longer. But if your dentist is forever suggesting crowns to cap your teeth, make sure you're not being "oversold," and find out why he has decided on the more expensive crowns instead of fillings.

Extraction happy dentists are not good dentists, so think twice before agreeing to an extraction, even if it's a wisdom tooth. Your mouth should feel comfortable and your bite should feel natural when the work is completed. Your gums should not bleed and you should be told how to take care of your teeth at home. If your dentist suggests expensive periodontal treatments, ask if there is a more conservative (and less expensive) approach, such as a gingival curettage for the removal of calculus and inflamed tissue.

Look out for the dentist who is constantly putting you off with temporary fillings. These mean extra visits for which he can charge more money. If you still feel pain after every dental visit, you're not getting quality dentistry. If your bridges get loose, or your dentures cause sore spots, or you can't chew properly, you're getting short changed. Don't be "oversold" on gold inlays, crowns, or replacement work unless you get another opinion. The dentist may be maximizing his own income at your expense. And look out for promises of cut-rate and assembly line dentistry. The quality generally suffers.

If you are not getting the quality dentistry you're paying for, you're throwing your money down the drain, and any fee you've paid is wasted. Every fee should reflect standards of good quality. If those standards are not upheld, you're not getting your dollar's worth.

---

*There are no guarantees. Just as a new tire can go flat, so can a new filling come out. Biting down too soon can cause this, and it doesn't necessarily indicate poor dentistry.

The Laws to Protect You

If a dentist overcharges you or mistreats you, your first step is to ask him to reconsider and make an adjustment. But if you cannot reach an agreement with him, you should be aware that there are *consumer laws* to protect you from fraudulent or incompetent dentists.

There are several federal laws which affect all retail credit in the United States, and these can provide certain guidelines for you in paying your bills. Your dentist is bound by the law to observe these rules, and there are penalties for breaking them. What are they? There are four you should know about.

1. The Federal Trade Commission's *Guides Against Debt Collection Deception* is complicated. But you should know that your dentist or his assistant cannot misrepresent to a delinquent patient who they are or why they are contacting him to obtain information. Subterfuge, such as pretending to be an attorney or credit rating office, is misrepresentation.
2. The Federal Communications Commission's *Public Notice on Use of Telephone for Debt Collection Purposes* clearly spells out invasion of privacy. Your dentist can phone you about an overdue bill, but violations such as calling your friends, employers, or neighbors are forbidden. Threatening calls, or calls falsely asserting your credit rating will be hurt are also violations. If your bill is overdue, your dentist or his assistant has the right to call at reasonable hours to discuss payment, but not to harass you.
3. "Regulation Z" of the Truth-in-Lending Law concerns credit. If you and your dentist agree upon payment in *more than four installments,* this law is applicable. It requires a written disclosure of all pertinent information regardless of whether or not a finance charge exists. However, it is *not* applicable if you decide, on your own, to pay in installments or whenever convenient.
4. The Fair Credit Reporting Act is probably one of the best consumer protection laws, because it really gives you a fighting chance to correct your records against unreasonable denial of credit. It says that if you are denied credit based on an adverse credit report from a credit agency, you must be

given the name and address of the agency. Your dentist must tell you that information, and he cannot hide behind an undisclosed "they" who denied your credit rating.

If you are aware of these laws, you are in a better position to handle the way you will pay your dental bills. You have a right to every protection of the law.

If, after exhausting every possible avenue for agreement, your dentist still has not satisfied you, you can report him to your local dental society. They will consider the case and make a recommendation. If your dental work is covered by insurance and you think you've been mistreated, you should consult the insurance company. The last resort is to consult an attorney. But it is wiser to exhaust every other possible means of adjustment first.

Anatomy of a Fee

Some patients believe there is only one correct treatment for any dental problem and only one fee established for it. On the contrary, a dental problem can be "correctly" treated in a variety of ways and with a variety of fees. Different patients who suffer *with the same complaint* may get different treatments, and you as a dental consumer should be aware of the wide spectrum of treatments and fees. You can influence your dentist's decision to choose one particular treatment over another, and the fee you pay may be the result of your own choices: the dentist you select; the questions you ask; the alternatives you explore. Your awareness as a dental consumer *can help to establish the fee you pay.*

Let's set up a case history of one hypothetical patient, Emily R., who will go to three different dentists with the same problem. Let's compare her experiences, the treatments she receives, and the fees she is charged. You will see three different approaches to the same problem (*all acceptable*), and fees from $50 to $5000.

The Patient

Emily R. is a 49 year old cafeteria worker in the local elementary school. She has not visited a dentist for three years. Fear of pain and high dental bills have delayed her visits. Now she must see a dentist at once because her face is swollen and she has a toothache which has kept her up for two nights. Emily's husband works as a car assembler in a regional plant. They have one daughter who is a senior in high school and plans to attend the local junior college while holding down a part-time job. Emily has six teeth in the upper jaw and seven in the lower. She wears a partial, upper, removable denture and a partial, lower, removable denture. She says, "I've never really been comfortable with these teeth, but I get along okay." Her partials were made ten years ago.

Case History No. 1: Dr. A

Emily's toothache has prompted her to check the telephone book for a dentist nearby. She calls Dr. A's office two blocks away and is told to come right over. The office is located on a main street over a pharmacy. The waiting room is small and dingy, with a light bulb missing from the overhead fixture and magazines a year old.

Dr. A, about 60, wears a white starched gown. He has a two-chair office and one dental assistant who writes down Emily's name and address and ushers her into the dental chair. Dr. A gives Emily a quick exam and says, "Your tooth is abscessed and has to come out. The remaining teeth don't look too good either. Have you ever considered having them all out?"

While Emily considers the question, Dr. A X rays the offending tooth and confirms that it has to be extracted. Emily is ashamed of the condition of her teeth. She agrees. "Okay. It's a good idea to get it over with. What would it cost?" Dr. A explains he will make immediate dentures; that is, take out all the remaining teeth and insert dentures the same day for $250 per denture. He also charges $10 for each extraction, times 13 teeth adding another $130. Total: $630. He further explains that immediate dentures usually "loosen up" after the gums "shrink" and Emily will need another set of teeth in about six months, adding another $500 to the $630. Grand total: $1130. Emily feels pressured to make a decision right away, so she consents to have the painful tooth removed and she will return in one week to start work on her immediate dentures.

The following day, Emily discusses the episode with her sister-in-law who had immediate dentures made two years ago. She advises Emily that a second set of dentures in six months is unnecessary. "Get the first ones relined like I did. Cost me only $150 for both, not $500. Save yourself $350, Emily."

When Emily returns to Dr. A's office, she asks him about relining dentures instead of getting a second set. "It could be done that way, but it's not the best way," he says. Dr. A takes several more X rays of the remaining teeth. He asks Emily to hold the film with her fingers and he doesn't bother with a lead bib. He tells Emily he requires a $200 deposit and the balance in full when the work is completed. "My fee includes three free adjustments, but if you need more, it'll be $10 extra." When Emily again brings up the relining question, he says, "We don't have to cross that bridge now."

(Summary of Dr. A's Treatment and Fees) Emily will have an immediate full upper and lower denture for $630, including 13 extractions and 3 adjustments. She may need another set of dentures in six months adding $500. Total? Perhaps $1130. No alternate treatment plan is presented.

Case History No. 2: Dr. B

The following case history describes the events that might occur if Emily selects Dr. B. We have the same patient, with the same dental problem.

Emily calls Dr. B's office and the secretary advises her that they will work her in as an emergency patient at 4:15. On arrival, Emily notes the office is crowded, waits 45 minutes, and at 5:00 is seated in the dental chair. Fifteen minutes later, Dr. B enters and listens briefly to Emily's complaint. Emily also expresses anxiety about spending a lot of money because her daughter will soon be going to college.

Dr. B examines her and says, "The tooth's abscessed." He confirms it with an X ray. "Better have it out," he says. "I can probably save your old partial and just add an artificial tooth to the plate. The extraction and denture repair will come to $50."

Emily is relieved that it will cost only $50. "Okay. Whatever you say, Doc."

(Summary of Dr. B's Treatment and Fees) Emily's abscessed tooth is extracted and a new tooth is added to her ten year old uncomfortable partial denture. She has spent only $50.

Case History No. 3: Dr. C

The third case history describes the treatment and fees if Emily had selected Dr. C. Again, we have the same patient with the same dental problem.

Emily phones Dr. C's office after checking carefully with two neighbors who had extensive work there. Both give Dr. C an excellent recommendation. Dr. C's secretary promises to work Emily in about 3:00 that afternoon. On arrival, Emily is asked to fill out a detailed medical-dental history. The waiting room is clean and inviting and she notices three dentist's names on the door. The office seems to hum efficiently.

In a little while a young dental assistant ushers her into a dental chair and tells her, "Dr. C will be right in. Don't worry, he'll get you comfortable in no time."

Dr. C, about 35, enters in a powder blue gown and studies the dental history while chatting briefly with Emily to break down her anxiety. After a thorough examination, he calls his hygienist to take X rays of the entire mouth. The dental hygienist places a lead bib on Emily as an extra precaution and each film is placed in a plastic film holder. Next, Emily is taken to another room where a large motorized Panorex X ray rotates around her head, scanning all her teeth, jaw bones, and sinuses. Then she is reseated in the operatory and Dr. C returns.

He has studied Emily's X rays and says, "There are several ways to treat you. The painful tooth is abscessed, *but that doesn't mean it has to come out.* We can save it. Your other teeth need work, too, but let's treat the painful tooth first and get you comfortable. Then we'll set up another appointment to discuss several plans when you're not under pressure."

Dr. C calls in his associate, Dr. D, and after a brief consultation, Dr. C explains that Dr. D will start root canal treatment and put a sedative inside the tooth. If Emily has any more pain, she is told to call their answering service, where the doctors can be reached 24 hours a day. He writes a prescription for pain in case she is troubled at night, and reassures her that this is a routine procedure. Emily is now free of pain and makes another appointment for a week later. Cost to date: $50 for treatment and X rays.

Dr. D's prediction is accurate and Emily has a painless week. At her next appointment, Dr. C puts her at ease and she thanks him for making her feel better and saving the tooth. Dr. C explains three different plans he has drawn up, contingent upon her study models.

(Treatment Plan 1) "I can extract your tooth and add an artificial tooth to your old partial, then clean and fill the remaining teeth that need work. This plan is not the one I'd recommend, but it will cost the least, about $85.

I'd rather save your tooth with root canal and still use the same old partial. That would cost $150 more for the root canal work. In other words, we'd save your tooth, and use your same partial. That will cost $150 for root canal and $35 for cleaning and filling. Total: $185. But you'd be saving your tooth."

(Treatment Plan 2) "An even better plan is to save the tooth with root canal therapy, fill the others, do some gum work and make two new partials. This plan would cost $600 for both new partials and $200 for the gum work, or an additional $800. Total: $985. It's more expensive, but it will give you more comfort than your old partials. And with the gum work and six month checkups, you'll probably enjoy the new partials for many, many years."

(Treatment Plan 3) The final plan Dr. C suggests is what he calls "total mouth rehabilitation." It is the most comprehensive and expensive of the three plans. Dr. C outlines a gingivectomy (gum surgery) and suggests crowns for the remaining teeth. Unlike the partial dentures which come in and out of the mouth, these restorations are permanently cemented in, so Emily will not have to remove and clean them every day. The results would be the best restorations

that modern dentistry can offer. "You'll feel better, look better, and be so much more comfortable."

"What would all this cost?" Emily asks.

Dr. C breaks down the fees for her. "The gingivectomy will be $350. You'll need 20 units of crown and bridge work at $225 each, or $4500. Total additional expenses: $4850."

"But, Doctor, if we add $150 for the root canal, that makes $5000. I can't afford $5000, Doctor. But I'd like to save the tooth, so let's do the root canal work and let me think about the rest of it. That's a lot of money."

Dr. C agrees. "Good idea. Think it over. At least now you understand the ways we can approach this. You can get from one place to another in a Volkswagon or a Cadillac. You've got to decide what you feel is best for yourself." He pauses. "Do you or your husband have any dental insurance through your jobs?"

"Insurance? I don't, but I'll check with my husband. Come to think of it, he's got some kind of policy at work."

"Bring it in and my secretary can help you."

When Emily returns for her next visit she still has not made up her mind. She brings her husband's insurance policy and asks Dr. C a lot of questions.

"Will this work hurt?"

"How long will the whole treatment take?"

"Can I pay it off, and how much deposit would you want on the $5000?"

"How long would the mouth rehabilitation last?"

"Will my husband's insurance cover any of it?"

Dr. C answers her questions clearly and directly. No, it won't hurt, only some minor discomfort now and then. The whole treatment could take about four months and appointments will average once a week for an hour or longer. Yes, you can pay off the bill over six months. No one can guarantee how long anything will last, but with good home care and regular checkups, your work could last a lifetime.

"And here's some good news. My secretary has read the policy and you're covered for $500 in any calendar year. Since this is November, we can submit a bill for root canal, X rays, and gum work this year, then legitimately collect another $500 in January. This will reduce your cost by $1000, leaving a $4000 balance. If you can put $2000 down, you can pay off the other $2000."

"Look," Emily says, "I'm 49 years old and I've never spent any money on myself. No vacations, no luxuries, nothing. I was planning to buy a new car, but I guess we can get along with the old one. I'd much rather put the money into myself to fix up my mouth than spend it on a car. They're both about the same price."

(Summary of Dr. C's Treatment and Fees) Emily has successful mouth rehabilitation. Her original painful tooth is saved through root canal work (cost: $150). She has a gingivectomy to restore her gums and save her teeth (cost: $350). And she has permanent crowns made for the remaining teeth (cost: $225 × 20 = $4500). Total: $5000. During the months of dental treatment, Emily becomes an informed dental consumer. She looks better, feels better, and her smile is radiant. She enjoys the added benefits of a tremendous psychological lift. She has paid a lot of money and she has received first class dentistry.

DISCUSSION

The fictitious Emily went to three different dentists with the same problem. **Dr. A** *offered to take out all of her teeth and give her dentures? Cost? $630 to $1130.* **Dr. B** *offered the cheapest stop-gap remedy of extracting the painful tooth and repairing her ten year old partials. Cost? $50.* **Dr. C** *is the only dentist who offered Emily any options. He suggested three different plans, outlining their benefits and liabilities. The costs ranged from $85 to $5000. Here we see the same patient, with the same dental problem, confronted with fees ranging from $50 to $5000. If you were Emily, what would you do?*

Obviously, not only do dentists differ in their fees and treatments, but so do patients in their ability to pay. Nevertheless, if you don't understand all the options available to you, you've been cheated out of a choice. Don't let anyone but you make the final choice. For some patients, Dr. A's treatment may have been best; for others, Dr. B's. But Dr. C was the *only* dentist who allowed Emily to decide, and her pocketbook was not the only factor in that decision.

Remember, the important thing is that fees and treatments vary. So consider your options, not just the fee.

Ann Landers, the syndicated columnist, printed a letter from an unhappy woman who described her own experience.

> *Haven't you read the ads or been in a drugstore lately? How could you fail to see the dozens of adhesive agents – powders, pastes, and liners for sale – all promising to help make dentures stick?*
>
> *Sure some dentures are fine, but a great many are not. I've spent over $3000 trying to get dentures I can eat with and I'm not exactly rolling in money. I had to go without necessities to pay those dental bills. I finally gave up last year after consulting a professor of dentistry at a well known university. I don't have much to laugh about these days, but when I do laugh, my uppers fall down. I'd give my right arm to have my own teeth back again. A good dentist can do a lot to save natural teeth. Mine didn't even try. He said, 'You'll be better off with dentures. They're cheaper, too.' Funny how people hate to spend money on their teeth – until it's too late. Then they'll spend a fortune on plastic ones that slide around, make sores and cause nothing but trouble.*
>
> (signed) Another Witness

Emily could have written this letter.

6
Tips on How to Preserve Your Teeth and Lower Your Dental Bills

Everyone knows that if you neglect your teeth, you're going to wind up with a mouth full of dental problems. This means going to the dentist to have him repair the damage. And that translates into spending a lot of money on dental bills.

You can do a great deal to save your money and keep those bills down by practicing preventive dentistry at home. Sure your dentist can instruct you about proper home care, effective hygiene, and good nutrition. But if all your fine resolutions go out the window, you're going to wind up with repair bills for a neglected mouth which can take an enormous chunk out of your budget. You can also wind up with false teeth and an appearance that adds 10 or 15 years to your age.

People who lay out thousands of dollars to buy a new car generally make it their business to see that it gets regular checkups. They are determined to protect their investment and avoid high repair bills. Obviously a car can be replaced. You expect to buy a new one after so many miles. *But you have only one set of teeth to take you through your entire lifetime!* So why not protect them and avoid the consequences of neglect?

Sharks Get Free Dentures

Unlike humans, sharks have many sets of teeth. As one set loosens up, it is replaced by an additional set. Nature provides the shark continuously with free dentures.

You can save thousands of dollars over your lifetime, perhaps enough to buy at least one new car, if you learn to be your own dentist at home every day. Here's how.

Home Care

Brush your teeth every day, if possible after every meal, and *at least every morning and night.* Don't scrub horizontally across the teeth. There are many acceptable methods of brushing your teeth. One is to *brush the way the teeth grow: up and down.*

Most of us don't carry a toothbrush around with us to brush after meals. So if you have dinner at a restaurant and can't brush, at least swish with water. This can dislodge the food particles that cling to your teeth and gums. You can swish with water and spit (if you can excuse yourself to the rest room), or simply swish and swallow (behind a napkin) at your seat.

Many cavities start at the gumline, so when you brush, get in between the teeth and get right to the gumline area where cavities can start. If you get the food out, you're doing a good job. The longer food collects after a meal the worse it is, so get to it quickly.

Toothbrushes

Don't use a hard brush and scrub until your gums bleed. Use a soft to medium brush, and brush gently. Natural bristles are kinder to teeth than nylon, but they take longer to dry (about 24 hours), so you should buy several. A straight handle with 3-4 rows can work well for you if you brush properly. Throw out that worn toothbrush. The bristles become misshapen and can scratch your mouth tissue. Also, you're apt to brush harder and irritate your gums.

Electric Toothbrushes

They're a boon to the handicapped or the lazy. But you can do just as well manually. Their main advantage is that all you have to do is apply the brush to different areas of your teeth. Although it's a gimmick, if the novelty of it encourages you to brush more often, it's probably worth the investment.

> **LBJ Invests Heavily in Electric Toothbrushes**
>
> *President Lyndon B. Johnson was sold on electric toothbrushes. Doris Kearns, his biographer, reports that she received no less than 12 electric toothbrushes from him engraved with the presidential seal. "I give these toothbrushes to friends," LBJ told her, "for then I know that from now until the end of their days they will think of me first thing in the morning, and the last at night."*

Electric toothbrushes found acceptable by the American Dental Association are Broxodent, General Electric, J.C. Penny, Sunbeam Cordless, and Touch-Tronic.

Toothpastes

Dentifrices are available as pastes or powders, and are intended to keep your teeth clean, free of food debris, plaque, and stain. As a rule, the powders are usually more abrasive than the pastes, and abrasion can wear down the enamel. Fluorides in toothpaste will fight decay in children during the cavity prone years. The American Dental Association Council on Dental Therapeutics has endorsed these:

Colgate with Gardol Plus MFP Fluoride
Crest with Fluoristan Mint or Regular Flavor
Macleans Fluoride

However, one wonders how the research that "proves" these products superior was arrived at, since the tests were funded by the manufacturers. Gleem II, which also contains fluoride, appears favorable too, but is not yet A.D.A. accepted. It is interesting to note that Gleem and Crest are not really competitive since they are both manufactured by Proctor and Gamble. In any case, it is the *act of brushing,* the mechanical dislodging of food debris, more than the choice of toothpaste, that does the most good.

What's in your toothpaste? Most contain abrasives, flavoring agents, and foaming agents. The flavors are varied, but the sweetener is usually saccharine. A few, like Calox Tooth Powder, use SUGAR! Most of us pick a toothpaste by the flavor and image the ad men sell us.* How much does that cost us? Americans spend $300 million a year on toothpaste!

Toothpastes that advertise they will whiten your teeth, increase your sex appeal, and get you a date or a wife are pandering to the lowest common denominator. Don't be taken in by the TV ads. Toothpastes can help to keep your mouth clean, but they are not guarantees of a cavity-free mouth, despite the "Look, Ma, no cavities!" PR job that Madison Avenue hucksters foist upon you. It's the toothbrushing that does the important work, not the dentifrice.

If your teeth are especially sensitive to cold or heat, there are commercial desensitizing toothpastes available at your pharmacy or supermarket. Ask your dentist about them. He may suggest you try Thermodent, Sensodyne, or Protect.

Sensitive to Hot or Cold? You're not Alone

Tooth hypersensitivity is a lot more common than most people believe. It is estimated that over 23 million people suffer from tooth hypersensitivity — or about one out of every seven patients. Over age 35? The number increases.

Irrigating Devices

Recently, the interdental water pick has become popular with patients who have periodontal disease and those who wear braces. How do they work? The water picks clean the teeth by irrigation with tiny jets of water that flush out food particles from difficult-to-reach spots where food collects. You can get the electric irrigator or the faucet irrigator type. But remember, they don't remove plaque, only food.

Patients with bridgework sometimes like the water pick because it can get under and around areas the toothbrush can't. On the other hand, some dentists don't like it because they feel it might do more harm than good. So all in all, it might be wiser not to invest in a water pick unless your dentist gives it the okay, especially in periodontal cases where the force of the water jet could further aggravate the

*The Council does *not* classify toothpastes without Fluoride (non-therapeutic).

gums. If you get the okay, use warm water and medium pressure, and use the pick under the guidance of your dentist who understands the unique circumstances of your mouth.

You might try the faucet type first because it's cheaper (about $8) before you invest in an electric one (about $25). The electric water picks acceptable to the A.D.A. are: Dento-Spray, Hydro-Dent, and Pulsar.

Mouthwashes

Halitosis?

"Even his best friend wouldn't tell him!"

Americans fork over the counter millions of dollars on breath sweeteners, mouthwashes, gargles, candy mints, toothpastes with mouthwash, and lozenges. Almost anything that promises fresher breath (whatever that is) can separate us from our money. Why? We seem to have an obsession about smelling bad. And the TV and magazine ads deluge us with promises of all sorts of pleasures *if only we avoid bad breath.* True?

No toothpaste, lozenge, or mouthwash can cure bad breath. All they can do is mask the foul odor. These medicated liquids are more cosmetic than therapeutic, and they will *not* prevent or cure sore throats, mouth disease, gum inflammation, or decay — any more than perfume will kill unpleasant body odor or illness. All they can do is give you the temporary feeling of "fresher breath." Look out for mint fresheners which contain sugar. You're only adding fuel to the fire when you constantly suck on them.

A Seedy Mouthwash

The cardamom seed is widely used in the Orient to sweeten the breath. At plush European cocktail lounges, it is offered as a breath mint after drinks much the way candy mints are offered to us in restaurants.

What do the experts think of mouthwashes? Dr. John Adriani, for years chief of the American Medical Association's Council on Drugs, says mouthwashes "destroy the necessary flora (bacteria) in the mouth, and mouthwashes may cause serious and permanent side reactions when used daily over protracted periods of time."

Lewis Josephs, American Dental Association manager of media relations, says, "All mouthwashes have been found to be unacceptable by the American Dental Association as aids to oral hygiene." He thinks they could do more harm than good.

Most mouthwashes contain alcohol which could cause drying of the mucous membrane. Below are a few tested in 1974 for alcohol content.

Listerine	25%
Micrin	20%
Scope	18.5%
Colgate 100	14%
Lavoris	5%

The FDA has classified Listerine containing boric acid and Lavoris containing Red No. 2 as unsafe.

The United States Federal Trade Commission recently ordered ads for Listerine to be corrected because it is *not* germicidal and will *not* prevent or cure colds or sore throats. Listerine is reported to reap 40% of the $275 million a year mouthwash market.

Persistent bad breath (not the kind that results from a feast of garlic, salami, and pickle) may be a sign of a more serious medical or dental problem. Chronic halitosis could be the result of infected tonsils, postnasal drip, digestive problems, diabetes, or decayed teeth, and should be checked.

The cheapest and safest mouthwash around is right in your own kitchen. And it won't cost you a nickel: *warm water and salt.* Don't throw your money out on commercial products. They're unnecessary, possibly harmful, and only serve to enrich the companies that manufacture them.

Dental Floss

The best mechanical aid to your toothbrush is dental tape or dental floss. Dental floss is easier to use and more popular. It's a strong thread (waxed or unwaxed) that passes between the teeth to remove the debris wedged there and along the gumline that your toothbrush missed. Flossing and brushing after the use of disclosing tablets are a powerful combination contributing to your oral hygiene. A clean mouth discourages plaque, the single most powerful cause of damage to your mouth.

How do you use it? Easy. Stretch the floss taut between the fingers of your right and left hands and then drag the thread between the teeth, up and down against the sides of the teeth, then across the gum line. Don't snap it and cut into your gums until they bleed. Do it gently, as if you are shining shoes. Waxed floss is a little easier to use if you have tight contact points, but many dentists prefer the unwaxed. There's a new floss on the market called Super Floss. It has a stiff section for threading under a bridge, a thicker spongy section in the middle, and a section of the usual unwaxed floss. You may find it easier to use.

If you have difficulty, there are floss threaders that can help you get under a bridge or into a hard to reach spot. There are even toothbrush-floss holder combinations, but they may be unwieldy, especially if they're made of sharp plastic. Flossing properly by hand is the greatest single adjunct to good toothbrushing. Try it until you get the hang of it and make it a regular part of your oral hygiene.

Toothpicks

A toothpick can be a lifesaver if you've just finished a steak and can't reach that maddening spot. A soft, flat, wooden toothpick, *not* a bobby pin or sharp instrument, can free the debris stuck between your teeth and make you feel instantly more comfortable.

Gum stimulators or stimudents are variations on the toothpick. They look like triangular toothpicks, are made of soft balsa-like wood, and come in packages of a dozen or 50, like a matchbook. They're handier than the rubber tip on the end of a toothbrush, and you can easily carry them around with you. They serve to massage the gums and are nicely flavored, so some people prefer them to toothpicks.

Denture Adhesives

As a temporary agent during the initial period of adjustment, these powders and pastes may be helpful. Mixed with water, they swell, become sticky, and help keep your dentures in place. But they should be discouraged as a permanent agent.* They can retain odors and encourage you to hang on to an ill-fitting denture that *can* cause sore spots and growths. Don't buy a home-relining kit either. If your denture is slipping and sliding around, spend the money on a visit to the dentist. It's a wise investment.

> **No Denture Adhesives At 93**
>
> *Alice Roosevelt Longworth, still feisty at the age of 93, is happy to display a mouthful of Roosevelt teeth. "These are natural," she likes to boast, "not store-bought."*

Denture Cleaners

Soaking dentures for 15 minutes doesn't always work, in spite of the elaborate claims on TV. Dentures should be scrubbed with a denture brush over a water filled basin, so if you drop them, they'll be cushioned by the water. You can buy a denture brush or use a good fingernail brush with ordinary soap. A long test tube or bottle brush works well for cleaning the inside of the clasps of removable partial dentures.

There are also ultrasonic denture cleaning devices which clean by ultra high frequency sound waves, about 20,000 cycles per second, but even here all the stain and debris cannot be removed without some brushing. The Branson Ultrasonic, E/MC Ultrasonic, and the Schick Ultrasonic seem to be the most effective.

> **The Ultimate Dental Shop**
>
> *Hans de Vos Klootwijk has opened the newest kind of shop in Hague, Netherlands. He and his wife sell dental products exclusively, from disclosing tablets to an international line of toothbrushes. An added feature is that instruction and preventive health clinics are provided at no extra cost for their customers and for patients sent by dentists.*

---

*Those acceptable to the A.D.A. are: Benefit Denture Adhesive, Co-Re-Ga Denture Adhesive Powder, Firmdent, Orahesive, Perma-Grip Denture Adhesive Powder, Wernet's Adhesive Cream, Wernet's Powder with Neoseal, and Super Wernet's Denture Adhesive.

Mouth Protectors

If you or your children play hockey, football, box, or engage in a potentially dangerous sport, wear a mouth protector and face guard *at every practice*. Properly fitted mouthguards can prevent nearly all injuries to the teeth and mouth. Warn your children, too, about practical jokers who come up behind them at the school water fountain and bang their faces down. Make sure you and your car passengers wear seat belts in case you must stop short.

When Jason Robards, Jr., the famous Broadway and movie star, smashed up his face in a car accident, he remembered "spitting something out and looking at it. It was my lip." Three operations and $45,000 later, Robards admitted he hadn't bothered to snap on his seat belt.

Emergency Care

Suppose you're on vacation and you suddenly develop a terrible toothache. You can't find a dentist. What can you do? Try a dental school or the emergency ward of a hospital.

In the meantime, avoid hot and cold and swallow two aspirin for relief of pain. *Don't* lay the aspirin against the tooth. You may also get some temporary relief by applying a cotton pellet soaked in oil of cloves into the cavity of the tooth (*not* on the mouth tissue). Sometimes a "sinus" toothache can be relieved by a decongestant. Sore gums may respond to a mouthwash of equal parts of 3% hydrogen peroxide (or sodium perborate) and warm water. But these are only temporary stopgap measures until you can reach the dentist.

If you've burned the roof of your mouth on hot pizza or soup, a mouthwash of one teaspoon of baking soda to a glass of water may ease the pain. And if you enjoy long hours of sunbathing when you're on vacation, and you're susceptible to cold sores on the lips, apply a layer of zinc oxide ointment over your lips before you stretch out.

A toothache is a universally understood pain. If you're in a foreign country and don't speak the language, sign language along with a few howls usually gets the message across. A dental first aid kit packed for emergencies could tide you over until you find a dentist. Pack oil of cloves, zinc oxide ointment, 3% hydrogen peroxide, aspirin or

Tylenol, and cotton pellets. It doesn't take up much room and it could save you a bleak day in a hotel room.

Overcoming Fears

"I'm scared to death of the dentist. What can I do?"

Most people are fearful and anxious about going to the dentist. The stereotype of a gleeful, sadistic man holding a whizzing drill over his patient, is perpetuated in comic strips, cartoons, and TV shows. Is it true? It's about as accurate as any other stereotype. Still, it persists. And the anticipation of pain produces increased fear.

> **Fear of Fillings**
>
> *Millions of people won't go to the dentist for necessary dental work out of fear of the dentist. How many? Estimates run around 10 to 12 million.*

Often, adults who are afraid of the dentist had an early childhood experience which conditioned them to believe that every dental contact would cause them intense pain. That is certainly *not* true. Still, "Will it hurt, Doc?" is probably the question most often asked.

Today's dentistry is nearly pain-free, and the painless dentist is more prevalent than the horrendous comic strip character. Modern anesthetics, analgesics, sophisticated high-speed drills with water sprays, and precision instruments make most dental procedures virtually painless. Unfortunately, you can know all that and *still* freeze up the minute you walk into the waiting room. If you are very apprehensive, ask your dentist for a topical anesthetic before a shot, or ask for a premedication pill. Of course, if your first experience when you were a child was to be dragged screaming into the dental chair, hand held to a swollen face and abscessed tooth, it's pretty difficult to erase the fear-riddled conditioning. What can you do about fears?

You could start by leveling with your dentist. Tell him straight out how frightened you are. If you've chosen a sympathetic fellow, he'll do everything to make you comfortable and allay your fears.

He'll even "prove" that he won't hurt. A sympathetic and sensitive dentist can do wonders to inspire your confidence. After a few painless visits, you'll probably go to him with less anxiety. And that is how reconditioning occurs.

Some people are afraid to get on a plane. They've tried everything — hypnosis, pills, even psychoanalysis — and they finally resort to behavior modification. There are films and cassettes on the subject which can be used in conjunction with psychological guidance. Try to modify your own behavior. You *can* overcome those fears by reconditioning yourself.

Ann Landers' answer to a young woman whose fiance had "awful gaps in his mouth" because he was riddled with fears was: "Most people who go around in need of dental care are afraid of pain. They don't realize that modern dentistry has changed a lot in the past 20 years." She also comments: "An unhealthy mouth means an unhealthy person."

Nutrition

If you eat correctly, you can save your health and your teeth. A basic principle of good diet is to *increase* the quantity of natural foods and *cut down on* refined and processed foods.

Raw vegetables (celery and carrots) and raw fruits (apples) are natural cleansers of the teeth and also serve to massage the gums. As nutrients, they are rich in vitamins and minerals. Unlike refined foods (white bread), they also contain cellulose, the bulk that is necessary to avoid the constipation and hemorrhoids that cost Americans millions of dollars for laxatives. These fibrous raw foods clean your intestines and release digestive enzymes which are lost when the food is cooked. They are an unbeatable combination: cleansing value plus food value plus bulk. Recent evidence seems to indicate that bulk added to your regular diet can also be a deterrent against cancer of the colon.

Vitamins

"If you eat a balanced diet," the Austin, Texas rancher insisted, "you don't need vitamins."

But who does? Many Americans skip breakfast, grab lunch on the run, and overeat at dinner. Then they snack all evening on junk foods, candy, cookies, and soda pop while watching their favorite TV shows. If that picture sounds like you, you *do* need vitamins and would probably profit from a daily vitamin supplement.

If you smoke, cigarettes take a heavy toll of Vitamin C. If you drink alcoholic beverages, a good B vitamin could help. And if you live the high pressure, stress ridden life, aggravated by urban pollution, vitamin E could be an advantage. A multivitamin once a day can make a difference in your overall health. Natural vitamin C (ascorbic acid) in the 500 milligram size taken with meals, plus vitamin E (for stress), has been touted as a powerful combination effective in prolonging life. A vitamin C deficiency can present the classic type of periodontal disease. Some people with gum problems have been helped by adding 2000 to 3000 milligrams of vitamin C daily to their diet. Check with your physician or dentist.

What To Avoid

Sugar! The worst junk and garbage foods are those containing white sugar: candy, soda pop, pastries, and cakes. Read the labels on packages before you spend a nickel, and watch out for additives and preservatives such as MSG. Most commercial meats are shot full of hormones and drugs. Cut down on meat as a source of protein and eat more fish, fowl, nuts, and beans which have less cholesterol. Replace the packaged sugar cereals with whole wheat cereals.

If you think all this is just another food fad, consider the case of the Hunza people (now part of West Pakistan), isolated for 2000 years, and having a natural diet containing no preservatives or white sugar. They lived to be over 100, fathered children at 90, and cancer, heart attacks, and high blood pressure were virtually unknown. Dr. Robert C. McCarrison, the British doctor who spent seven years with the Hunzas, noted the teeth of their children were perfect, with healthy gums. "They clean their teeth with little twigs . . . aided by a natural diet." They don't have Crest and they don't have dentists, but dental disease is non-existent. They must be doing something right!

As far as tooth decay is concerned, remember this:

SUGAR RUINS TEETH

So do easily fermentable carbohydrates. If you cut down on these, you can prevent the cavities that cause you those huge repair bills.

AVOID THESE	
soda pop	candy
ice cream	sweetened cereals
chocolate milk	pastas
imitation fruit juices	marshmallows
sweet sauces	cakes
white bread	cookies
jams	syrup
pies	molasses
canned fruits in heavy syrup	honey

You should replace those foods which destroy healthy teeth with raw fruits and vegetables which are natural detergents.

INCREASE THESE	
celery (raw)	apples
carrots (raw)	pears
lettuce	green peppers (raw)
cauliflower (raw)	plums
radishes	unsweetened juices
cantaloupes	nuts and seeds
oranges	

The kind of diet recommended by nutritionists for general health holds true for dental health. That means there is a strong relationship between diet, tooth decay and periodontal disease.

For adequate nutrition, you need to eat food from these four groups:

MILK GROUP: Milk, cheese, dairy products, yogurt
MEAT GROUP: Veal, beef, pork, lamb, fowl, fish, eggs, dry beans and peas, nuts
VEGETABLE-FRUIT GROUP: Raw is better than cooked. The dark green and yellow vegetables are mineral and vitamin rich.
BREAD-CEREAL GROUP: Choose the whole grain wheat, bran, and enriched ones.

A "Safer" Sugar

Wouldn't it be marvelous if you could eat all the candy you wanted without suffering any bad effects? Wouldn't it be great if someone would invent a delicious, sweet sugar that's not harmful to teeth? Well, it may be on the way. At the State University of New York at Stony Brook, Dr. Thomas F. McNamara has developed a "safer sugar." This preparation contains sucrose, along with two other sugars, fructose and maltose, and the *combination* appears to be *75% safer for teeth.* Care for a Mary Jane for dessert?

> **Hard to Limit Sweets? Even Harder to Limit Calories**
>
> *A woman who found it difficult to diet had her dentist wire her jaws together so she couldn't eat any solid food. Did she lose weight? Yes. But Dr. Daniel M. Laskin, editor of the Journal of Oral Surgery, warns that such gimmicks could be dangerous. What's foolproof? Proper motivation and establishing new eating habits.*

Mass Prevention of Cavities

In 1975, 300 to 325 seventh graders from Hartford and West Hartford, Connecticut began helping researchers at the University of Connecticut School of Dental Medicine to find an *anti-bacterial mouthrinse.* Supported by a $300,000 three year grant from the National Institute of Dental Research (NIDR), reports indicate research is under way to find a safe and effective agent. A wild dream? Dr. Stephen Kegeles says "means may be available shortly for the mass prevention of dental caries." The NIDR Caries Task Force predicts that enough knowledge now exists "to make this disease almost preventable by 1980."

Prevent Death By Choking

If you wear dentures, your sense of touch is diminished. So watch out for a foreign object such as a fish bone or chicken bone that can easily be swallowed. Death from partially chewed lobster or steak occurs at many business dinners every year. The causes? Poor teeth or poor dentures and one too many martinis!

If you see someone choking, grab him from behind with both hands and give him a sharp squeeze inward and upward above his waist to dislodge the object. You could save a life.

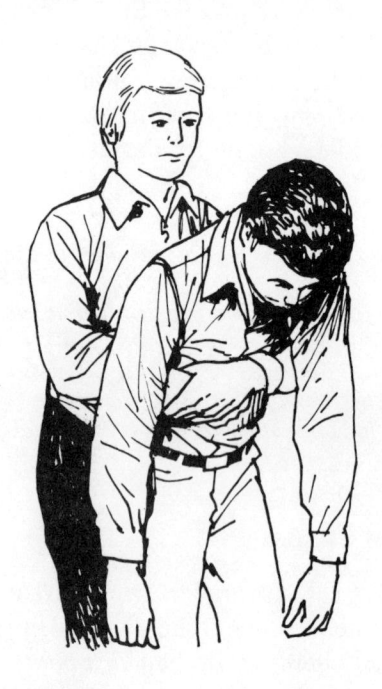

You Can Save the Life of a Choking Victim

If you are alone and choking, use your own fist to apply force below the diaphragm with a sharp inward and upward force.

Prevent Headaches

Grinding your teeth at night? That's one way to relieve inner conflicts, according to dental researchers Dr. William R. Cinotti and Dr. Arthur Grieder of the New Jersey College of Medicine and Dentistry. Bruxism, the term for this kind of grinding, can cause headaches, and about 10% of adults do it.

"Men get ulcers and heart attacks, and women grind their teeth," they report. 80% of the bruxers are women. If you're a bruxer, your dentist can help you by equilibrating your bite, or fitting you with a night guard or a bite plate.

Prevent Mouth Injuries

Do you bite off thread instead of using a scissors? Do you open bobby pins with your teeth? Bite hard candy? Crack nuts with your teeth? Use a pin to remove food stuck between your teeth? If you do, you can be chipping your teeth and causing hairline fractures in your fillings. That means larger repair bills to pay. So don't use your teeth as a tool and prevent injuries.

Pit and Fissure Sealants

"Tommy got something magic put on his teeth, and now he won't get any cavities, Daddy," the fourth grader reported.

Fluorides? No. Something relatively new. What is it? Does it work? What does it cost? Can it save you money?

Dr. Leon M. Silverstone of London reported plastic sealants can be highly effective in preventing children's cavities. The British doctor noted decay reduced as much as 90%, and effectiveness lasted as long as four years. Is there a hitch? Should your dentist be using plastic sealants on your children's teeth?

Some already do. But they can only be applied to the biting (occlusal) surfaces of the teeth and they don't reduce cavities on the other surfaces. Therefore, some dentists feel their use is limited. In addition, applying them properly takes time. So your dentist may charge you almost as much to protect the tooth as to fill it. Does it pay?

Right now it seems like a calculated risk. But if you're a gambling man or woman, ask your dentist how he feels about it. Then make up your own mind.

Motivation: It's Up To You

You already know how to keep your mouth clean. That's *Step One: Oral Hygiene.* And you know about *Step Two: Nutrition and Diet.*

You also know the importance of *Step Three: Regular Dental Checkups.* What's left? What else can you do to reduce dental disease and save money?

That's *Step Four: Motivation,* the ingredient that makes all the other steps work. You've got to be a partner in your own health care. Only *you* can do it. Do it for your health's sake. Do it for your wallet's sake.

If you become a partner, an active participant in preventing dental disease, you could save yourself and your family thousands of dollars in a single year. You can use those savings for the luxury items you feel you can't afford: that vacation you've been promising your wife; the new car you've been eyeing; the college tuition for your child or yourself.

Whose car would you rather buy? Your dentist's or your own?

CONSUMER TIPS TO SAVE YOUR TEETH AND YOUR WALLET

- Brush your teeth up and down and at the gumlines every morning and night. If you can't brush after every meal, swish to dislodge food. The longer food collects after a meal, the more damage it can cause.
- Throw out your worn toothbrush so that you don't irritate your gums with scraggly bristles.
- Toothpastes endorsed by the A.D.A. are Colgate with Gardol Plus MFP Fluoride, Macleans Fluoride, and Crest with Fluoristan Mint or Regular. Remember, it is the act of brushing more than the choice of toothpaste that does the most good. Brush!
- Don't invest in a water pick until you check with your dentist. In periodontal cases, it could do you more harm than good.
- Don't throw your money out on commercial mouthwashes. The cheapest and safest is right in your own kitchen — warm water and salt.
- Dental floss used properly every day is the single greatest adjunct to good toothbrushing and oral hygiene.
- Don't use denture adhesives or relining kits to hang on to an ill fitting denture that's causing sore spots. See your dentist if your denture doesn't fit.
- Scrub dentures with a brush over a water filled basin, so if you drop them they'll be cushioned from breaking.
- Prevent accidents by using car seatbelts. Use mouth protectors at every sports practice.
- If you are especially fearful, tell your dentist so he can give you some extra care: a topical anesthetic before a shot or a premedication pill.
- Raw vegetables and raw fruits are far better for you than refined and processed foods. They are also natural cleaners and detergents of the teeth, and they massage the gums.
- AVOID SUGAR. SUGAR RUINS TEETH. So do easily fermentable carbohydrates. Soda pop, candy, and pies are costing you money in dental repairs.
- If you wear dentures which decrease your sense of touch, beware of choking on a fish or a chicken bone.

- Headaches caused by grinding your teeth at night may be relieved by wearing a night guard or bite plate, or by having your bite balanced.
- The magic ingredients for good teeth and low dental bills are: *Oral Hygiene; Nutrition and Diet; Regular Dental Checkups;* and *Motivation.* Be a partner in your own home care and you can save thousands of dollars on dental repairs.

7
Dental Insurance Plans:
How to Get the Most Out of Your Policy

Dental insurance has been called "the hottest game in town." Why? What should you know about it? Where can you get it? What does it cost?

Almost everyone has some form of *medical* health insurance, but until recently, *dental* coverage was largely restricted in our country. Ten years ago, only about two out of a hundred Americans had any kind of coverage for paying their dental bills. In 1973, that figure rose to one in ten. Estimates for 1980 show that 60 million people will carry some form of plan (one out of four Americans will be covered). You could be one of them. What's it all about?

Virtually all dental insurance is written on a group, not an individual basis. Individual dental policies are around, but they are scarce and offer very restricted protection. But the group dental insurance is a prepaid plan that can pay a substantial part of your dental bill.

Most of the growth in dental insurance stemmed from three national contracts that included coverage for employees of the United Auto Workers (UAW), the United Steelworkers, and the Communication Workers of America. The A.T. & T. plan, which is less comprehensive than the UAW plan, covers minimal orthodontics and surgical periodontics in the benefit package, but preventive and diagnostic services are reimbursed at 100% of the *usual, customary, and reasonable charge,* called UCR. After a one time $50 deductible, there is an annual maximum allowance of $500 per person. The A.T. & T. package adds another 3.5 million Americans to the rapidly growing arena of dental insurance for Americans.

Dental payment plans are not unknown to other countries around the world. In West Germany, dental care is provided within the National Health Insurance System, to which 93% of the population belongs. The other 7% are either privately insured or have no insurance at all. The Norwegian government offers regular dental exams, topical fluorides, restorations, periodontal treatments, extractions, and oral surgery to school children who go to salaried dentists. In Japan, low cost dental care is provided through the national Social Security legislation which pays 50% of the costs for everyone except high income patients. In New Zealand, preschool and primary children receive dental care given by a special type of "school dental nurse" in their own school dental clinic. So dental insurance is not unknown.

Because dental insurance is new to most Americans, the unwary consumer can get bogged down in a morass of pitfalls, red tape, and misunderstanding. The vocabulary itself is confusing; a patient is faced with words like eligibility, deductibles, co-payments, prior authorization, and the gobbledegook of insurance forms. To say the least, it's frustrating. But you don't need a glossary of terms to get to the bottom of it and you can save a lot of money if you understand what it's all about.

Most people come to the dentist uninformed and vaguely aware, "Maybe my insurance will cover it." This can work against you and you can lose out if you don't understand your benefits. How do you find out?

Do You Have Dental Insurance?

If you think you have a *third party* payment plan (that means an insurance plan), FIND OUT. Maybe your union secretary or shop steward has informed you that you finally are getting "the plan" as a fringe benefit. Now it's up to you. Get a copy of the brochure which spells out what your coverage is, which members of your family are included, and what your benefits are. Your union or employer should furnish you with this information explaining how the plan works. Read it carefully until you understand clearly what you're entitled to.

Most dental insurance covers the employee and his family and includes a wide range of basic services. Your plan could include

X rays, prophylaxis, fillings, extractions, and periodontal treatments. Some dental insurance plans even cover dentures, fixed and removable bridges, and orthodontic care. Services that are not usually covered are hospitalization and purely cosmetic dentistry. But even if your *dental* insurance excludes hospitalization, check back on your *medical* insurance policy because hospital care and surgery may be included. You may be able to collect for dental work *done in a hospital under your medical insurance.*

Different Plans

There are basically two types of plans for dental insurance. One plan pays for dental care based on a *table of allowances.* This means there is a fee schedule for each dental procedure and an allowance the insurance company will pay for it, perhaps 75% of the scheduled amount, or 100%, or whatever. For example, let's say you have an initial exam for which your dentist charges $15. The table of allowances may set $10 for an initial exam and pay 100% of that $10. So you owe the dentist $5. Some programs pay *only a percentage of the table of allowances,* for example 75%. In that case, your insurance would cover 75% of the $10, or $7.50; then you owe the dentist the difference, another $7.50. Most dentists prefer to bill the patient for their fee, and they hold the patient responsible for that payment in full (the $15). But they will fill out the insurance forms so you can be reimbursed by the insurance company. However, if the insurance disallows the claim, you owe the dentist the full fee.

The UCR plan is the second type and stands for usual, customary, reasonable fee. This plan will pay a percentage of your dentist's UCR fee. Many plans pay 75% of the UCR fee, so under that plan you'd receive 75% of $15, or $11.25 toward your bill, and you'd owe your dentist only $3.75.

Deductibles, Limitations and Exclusions

Watch out for the small print. As the saying goes, the large print gives it to you and the small print takes it away. Some programs have a $50 deductible similar to automobile insurance. You pay the first $50, then the plan takes over. The deductible could be an annual or a one time only deductible.

Your coverage might also have a maximum amount payable for each person covered, say $600 per calendar year. You should know this because it could mean a saving of hundreds of dollars. Let's say your wife needs periodontal treatments, root canal work, and crowns. You are covered for these procedures up to $600 for each member of your family. You could begin her periodontal work and root canal therapy at the end of one calendar year, then start the crowns at the beginning of the next year, *maximizing your benefits to $1200*. If you didn't know the terms of your plan and had all her dental work completed in one calendar year, you would have spent an extra $600 unnecessarily.

You may have a "waiting period" before benefits begin, and there may be certain conditions to fulfill for eligibility. Get it all clear in your head *before* you begin treatment.

In some cases, the insurance companies require certification of eligibility and predetermination of benefits *before the work is done*. This means your dentist will submit a treatment plan to your carrier to determine how much the carrier will pay. It could take a few weeks, but then you'll know exactly how much will be paid and how much you'll have to spend out of your own pocket.

A recent* agreement representing 300 railroads, and covering 1.5 million employees and dependents in 14 national railroad unions, is representative of a typical insurance package. Prevention, basic, and emergency dental services are covered at 75% of UCR. Prosthetics, crowns, and gold restorations are payable at 50% of UCR. Orthodontic dental services will be covered at 50% with a lifetime maximum of $500. There is an annual $50 deductible per person and an annual maximum of $500 per person. The estimated cost of the program through 1977 is about $100 million. Understanding this benefit package can save a railroad worker and his family thousands of dollars in dental bills every year.

Reducing Insurance Hassles

Insurance forms are a pain in the neck to everyone — the patient, the dentist, and the third party. But since they are necessary, you can reduce the hassle if you handle the forms the right way. This will make it easier for everyone involved.

Your dentist is probably buried under a pile of forms: dental insurance forms, welfare forms, medicaid forms. As the paper work becomes heavier and more and more of his office time is spent "filling out forms," tempers can flare. Sometimes the dentist is upset because the carrier doesn't cover the *level* of treatment he prescribes. Dental insurance doesn't cover everything, only a portion of your dental bills. Often the insurance covers the *least* expensive treatment.

Dentists complain bitterly of daily frustrations with third party plans: long cumbersome forms, delays in approval and payments, poor communications, and disagreements about treatment plans. Obviously, the dentist doesn't want the carrier to tell him what to do, what treatment to choose, or how to go about his profession. Only the dentist and his patient can decide what's best. The insurance company, dentists feel, should stick to matters of coverage and benefits. Dentists rage that the irreconcilable disputes with carriers are the result of their interference with diagnosis and the doctor-patient relationship. They feel the insurance company oversteps its bounds and makes unfair inferences to the patient which puts them in a poor light.

The insurance companies, on the other hand, charge the dentist with all sorts of misdealings. They claim dentists coerce patients into expensive treatments, predate and postdate claim forms, pad the bills for extra services, and improperly label treatments to maximize benefits (such as calling a prophylaxis a subgingival curettage).

What can you do about it? Can any good come out of dental insurance plans? How can a dental consumer reduce the frustration and receive the benefits due him?

First of all, get a copy of the brochure that spells out your plan, and go over it so *you* know your benefits. If you are knowledgeable, you can help your dentist get the most out of your insurance. When you go to the dentist, don't be vague and confused about your insurance. Know your benefits.

Dental insurance is designed to take the sting out of dental bills, not to pay everything. So don't be suspicious that your dentist is cheating you just because his fee is higher than the insurance coverage. Ask about his fees for a particular procedure, then ask him to help you collect what is due you.

Dr. Frederick Harvey, President of the New Jersey Dental Society, said he once treated a patient, and charged his usual fee of $230. But the insurance company paid only $23.11 of that. He claims insurance payments are unrealistic in some cases and tend to mislead people into thinking that if the insurance only pays $23.11, that's what the dentist should have charged. He cautions that the "fine print" may give the company the right to pay for the least expensive alternative treatment *if the insurance company says it's adequate.* So although the insurance company can't force you to have a particular treatment, it may also pay for the least expensive type. The rest comes out of your pocket.

Like Dr. Harvey, many dentists resent "the dictatorship by insurance companies." Dr. L. M. Kennedy, past president of the American Dental Association, said, "...more than 90% of the problems confronting our profession today are either directly or indirectly related to the emergence of third party involvement in dental health care."

Although ultimately the dentist and you decide on your treatment, you should be aware that certain treatments your dentist recommends are *not* covered by insurance. So know what part of the fee is your responsibility.

Filling Out The Insurance Claim

Your dentist will help you prepare and file the claim form, but you can help him by filling out the personal part ahead of time: name, address, date of birth, social security number, etc. If you get all that done in advance, he'll appreciate it because you've saved him valuable office time. Patients who consume ten minutes looking up their social security number while the assistant steams do not endear themselves to the office, and get short shrift. So make it easy, and be accurate and complete in preparing the form.

Tell your dentist everything you know about your plan including exclusions, deductibles, etc. so he can maximize your coverage and see that you get every benefit to which you are legally entitled. *Tell him before your treatment begins.* Maybe *both* you and your spouse have insurance plans (called *dual coverage*). In California, where the dental plans are heaviest, about 15% of patients have this dual coverage. What can that mean to you? It means that both a primary and secondary insurance carrier are involved. Tell your dentist this. Let's say you are treated under your own insurance plan. Then your prime carrier pays the benefits. In a family with dependent children, the father's insurance company is usually considered the primary carrier and the mother's the secondary. Dual coverage cases can mean that the combined carriers will be responsible *for the entire fee.*

An efficient dental office usually designates one business assistant to handle all the dental forms that come in. The dentist will train a competent member of his staff, and give him or her the authority to fill out the forms, prepare pre-authorization information, submit X rays and data to the carriers, and follow up on payments and records. It's an enormous and demanding task full of code numbers, and it takes up a great deal of time. Although the business assistant may be able to advise you and explain aspects of your insurance, rely on yourself, too, and be clear about the facts of your own coverage.

Over 70% of dental offices have at least some insurance work. And that's on the upswing. More and more dental offices are getting involved with third party insurance forms, but that doesn't mean your dentist is an expert in the insurance field. Check with him, check with your place of employment or union office, and check with your carrier. If you become familiar with the terms of your insurance plan, you can utilize its benefits to the maximum and save yourself hundreds of dollars a year in dental bills.

Will your dentist charge you for filling out the claim forms? Most dentists do not, but a few do — anywhere from $2 to $7 after the first form, which is free. Some states are moving to outlaw any fee. In New Jersey, Governor Byrne signed into law Assembly Bill 1343 prohibiting any dentist or dental service corporation from charging an extra fee for completing a form for a health insurance claim. Check to see if such a fee is legal in your state if your dentist attempts to tack on a fee.

Advantages of Dental Insurance

The most apparent advantage of having dental insurance is that it saves you money. But as more and more patients are being covered by third party plans, other advantages are surfacing in addition to the financial benefits. What are they?

More people are going to the dentist and receiving necessary dental care. Obviously, if you have an insurance plan, you're more likely to go to the dentist, because you know the sting of paying the bill is going to be erased by your insurance company. So people are seeking treatment *more often,* and therefore getting better dental care. Dental neglect is less likely to occur among patients who have dental insurance plans and see their dentist.

> **Dental Neglect**
>
> *A study recently estimated that over a quarter of all Americans have never been to a dentist or have not seen a dentist in the last five years.*

It's interesting to observe, too, that more teeth are being saved and less removable prosthetic appliances are being made. There is more emphasis on endodontics, periodontics, and fixed prosthetics, and less on extractions. All this is in keeping with better dental health.

Prepayment plans are in their infancy and many are fraught with bureaucratic tangles within the various dental insurance packages. The daily frustrations still plague the dentist and patient alike. When dental insurance plans went into effect on the West coast, delays of three months were not unusual. But many of these problems are being wiped out.

One of the improvements is the use of the universal or uni-claim form that almost all dental insurance companies are now accepting. Instead of being confronted with a myriad of different company forms, the dentist can now submit one universal form, replacing the 250 different forms in use. Even if the patient brings in his own form, the dentist can staple it to the uni-claim form. That saves time, eliminates red tape, and reduces frazzled nerves.

The Delta Plans

Another outgrowth of the third party insurance plans are the Delta Plans. These are nonprofit corporations, formed by organized dentistry to compete against the nearly 100 commercial carriers. The

Delta Dental Plans arose as an alternative to commercial insurance plans which often infuriated the dentist.

Dr. Donald C. Meyer, a Bronx dentist, says, "These third-party payors are gaining increasing control over the health professions. They are dictating treatment, regulating fees, and creating a paperwork burden." He believes, "The third party payors are planting doubts in patients' minds about the quality of the health care they are getting and the integrity of their physicians and dentists." He has harsh words for the insurance companies. "They pick the least expensive treatment regardless of what is best for the patient. It's then up to the dentist to appeal. This is a time consuming procedure filled with red tape."

The Delta Plans are *run by dentists* and therefore eliminate the intrusion of the outsider (insurance carrier) into the dentist-patient relationship. Of the 30 million Americans now covered by dental insurance, the Delta systems cover about 11 million. This assures the private dentist's voice in dental insurance plans by offering *its own insurance,* which it says is more responsive to patients' needs.

The Delta Plans do not interfere with the plan of treatment you and your dentist decide on. However, if your dentist feels the decision on benefits is incorrect, he could ask for a further evaluation through *peer review,* a committee of dentists who report on their findings. Dentists feel this eliminates the intrusion of commercial insurance interests and safeguards the legitimate concerns of patients. After all, they say, who understands what patients need better than the dentist?

Dr. Joseph Pollack, president of the nonprofit New Jersey Dental Service Plan, sings the praises of the five year old Delta Plan. Employee groups can buy coverage, which pays the whole fee or some percentage. 90% of New Jersey dentists are participating. Dr. Pollack says that, for an extended treatment, a dentist must submit a predetermination claim, and *within five working days* the patient is notified how much the plan will pay. "This takes the guesswork out of it," he says. Dr. Pollack estimates the average family policy costs about $15 a month.

Shoes or Teeth

The average per capita spending for an American is $30 on his teeth – about the cost of a pair of shoes. This figure reflects a lack of dental attention rather than inexpensive dental fees.

Whether you have dental insurance through a commercial plan or a Delta Plan, you should know that it is the patient's responsibility to question all work done and all fees charged. Don't expect the plans to "look out for you" like some big Daddy who protects you against harm.

Get updated information on the plan your employer has provided. The coverage and benefits could change from year to year and you should be aware of any alterations in what's due you. If you think you are going to lose your job or change jobs, by all means get your dental work done *before your policy expires.* Get every advantage you're entitled to. And if you have the option of choosing a wage increase or a health insurance package, *you're probably better off with insurance.* Inflation and taxes can reduce that wage increase to a pittance, but the health insurance can go a long way for you and your family. If you become involved with a claim dispute, report it promptly to your employer group for negotiation with the carrier or the dental association's peer review committee.

Maybe your employer is considering a health insurance package. If so, get involved with the negotiations and help select the plan which will serve you and your family best. You can save a lot of money with dental insurance coverage, and plans vary considerably. If you call the shots as a representative, or you can influence your union representative, you'll have your say about choosing the right plan. When negotiating, if your group cannot afford total coverage, you can start with basic coverage and eventually add more comprehensive benefits that include bridgework and orthodontics.

National Health Insurance

At one time, some people were predicting that National Health Insurance was a shoo-in — that we'd have it for sure because its time had come. However, there appears to be a lot of flies in the ointment.

For one thing, dentists oppose it. Dr. Harold Hillenbrand, former executive director of the American Dental Association, feels opposition to any dental involvement in a national health plan stems from fear of government intervention in dental policy making. He thinks National Health Insurance will be beset with the same problems faced by Amtrak and the Postal Services, and could only result in a giant patchwork designed for political appeal. The running gag among dentists opposing a national plan is, "If you love the way your postal services operate, ask for National Health Insurance."

President Ford's veto of the National Child Health Protection Act seemed to underscore his administration's lack of concern for national health. If a National Health Insurance program does become a reality, then health care could become our country's largest industry. Whether we have the manpower and the womenpower to implement such a program under the present system is still being argued.

Right now, with President Carter at the helm we may get the first real effort to begin a national health program. However, realistically it could take four to five years of phasing in. And what it will include in *dental* care is still under siege. Many people like David Pittle, vice chairman of the United States Consumer Product Safety Commission, believe, "The consumer gets nothing for which he does not fight." He says the White House under Jimmy Carter "will be the most sympathetic (to consumers) in modern history."

Even if National Health Insurance does come to be, the inclusion of dental care is by no means certain. Of the dozens of proposals before Congress, comprehensive dental care for children to age 12 and dental care for the elderly seem to be a front runner. The New Zealand system that allows "dental nurses" to take over some of the routine services appears unlikely in the United States, although expanded roles for auxiliary are on the upswing. But the 94th Congress, torn with the problems of economic recession, seemed far from enacting any legislation for a national health care plan. And the rhetoric of the election rarely included such touchy issues.

No one seems to agree on one plan, and so we are no nearer a solution than before, when jealous health committees chopped up the case for National Health Insurance. The Health Security Act of 1975, coauthored by Senator Edward M. Kennedy (D-Mass.) and Representative James C. Corman (D-Calif.), offers dental care to all children to age 15, half of it paid by payroll taxes and the rest out of general revenues. But the issue of payroll taxes gets in the way. The American Dental Association is pushing its own plan, so nothing concrete has been arrived at.

In the meantime, dental health insurance plans are widely offered through commercial carriers and Delta Plans. More and more groups of employees are being covered, and it's likely that you, or a member of your family, may be included in such a plan. If so, you can probably get a lot of dental work done without turning your pockets inside out. And the more you know about the plan, the more money you can save. Being an informed dental consumer about your insurance can earn you hundreds of dollars in dental benefits. Find out what they are. Then get the best dentistry and let your insurance plan cover every benefit you're entitled to.

Malpractice Insurance

Malpractice insurance is what *your dentist pays* to insure himself against claims patients may make against him. *He* pays the premiums for it, so it might seem to you that you have no interest in it. Not so. If his rates go up, that will probably be reflected in higher fees to you. But fortunately, dental malpractice rates have not risen very much compared to medical malpractice rates.

In Southern California, some physicians are faced with a 327% increase in their malpractice insurance premiums. For a surgeon to operate on a patient in Los Angeles, he would have to pay $36,000 in insurance. The results have been catastrophic: physicians' strikes, personal agony, hospitals brought to a standstill, maybe even deaths.

Unlike medical insurance, the dentist's malpractice insurance rate, about $200, has not risen much over the years. Why? The most obvious reason is that there are rarely any large settlements, no loss of limbs or sight as in surgical malpractice cases, and no life-or-death cases. Even if a dental patient feels wronged (the wrong tooth was extracted) and he has explored every other avenue, engaging an attorney is not a simple procedure.

For one thing, the economic gains to an attorney will not be high. Given a case which might win a $5000 to $6000 settlement, the attorney might get one third (perhaps at most $2000), and out-of-pocket expenses for expert witnesses, duplication of records, etc. could run several thousand more. So in the end, there's not much left for the person to recover, or enough for the attorney to want to take the case.

A prominent New Jersey attorney who specializes in medical malpractice cases says the economics of dental malpractice cases preclude his taking them.

"Besides," he says, "there are two elements that must be present to make a malpractice case:

1. *Deviation* from accepted standards of good dental practice, and
2. Injury *caused* by number one."

Unless both are indisputably present, most attorneys won't take the case. So just because your daughter's orthodontia treatments didn't turn out exactly the way you envisioned it, that doesn't mean you have a case against your dentist.

Since dental settlements are neither high nor common, dental insurance rates haven't exploded like medical insurance rates. This means savings to you. As long as dental malpractice cases don't rise, your dentist's "overhead" won't be passed along to you in higher fees.

If you feel you were wronged, do explore every other possibility *before* engaging an attorney. Discuss your complaint first with your dentist. If you do not get satisfaction, go to your dental society, insurance carrier, or consumer advocate agency. If nothing else works, then consult your attorney.

Frivolous Malpractice Suit Boomerangs

A jury recently awarded Dr. Leonard Berlin, a 41 year old radiologist, $8000 in compensatory and punitive damages against the patient and her two attorneys who sued him. Why? They sued without reasonable cause. The patient sought $250,000 from Dr. Berlin and wound up paying him $8000. This precedent setting verdict carries an important message that discourages frivolous, non-meritorious cases against doctors. They can boomerang!

The patient's lawyer will appeal. "If it were allowed to stand," he warned, "no lawyer is going to want to take a case because they're afraid of being sued." He sounded almost like a doctor.

DENTAL INSURANCE CONSUMER TIPS

- Find out if you, or a member of your family, has dental insurance through your union or employer.
- Understand your benefits and know what you're covered for.
- Ask for your company's brochure that explains the plan. Then keep it handy for reference when you go to the dentist.
- Ask your dentist how to maximize your benefits to receive everything you're entitled to in a calendar year.
- Tell your dentist you have dental insurance *BEFORE* he starts work.
- Reduce insurance hassles by filling out the personal part of the insurance form ahead of time. Be accurate and complete and you'll avoid delays in payment.
- If you and your spouse both have insurance plans (dual coverage), both carriers together could pay the entire fee.
- If your state prohibits a fee for filling out dental insurance forms, make sure your dentist doesn't tack on a fee.
- Investigate the advantages of the Delta Plans sponsored as non-profit dentist-run plans, which compete against the commercial carriers.
- If you are going to leave your job or change jobs, get your dental work done before your policy expires.
- You're probably better off choosing a health insurance package than a raise, which can be reduced to a pittance after inflation and taxes.
- If you believe you have been wronged by your dentist, explore every avenue you can (complaints to your dentist, the local dental society, your insurance carrier, your consumer advocate agency) *before* you engage an attorney.

8
Taking the Mystery Out of "The Dontias"

The famous humorist Will Rogers once said, "Everybody is ignorant, only in different subjects."

Many professions, especially law and medicine, are shrouded in a thick cloud of mystery and technical language. This acts as a barrier between the professional, *the knowing one,* and the layman, *the ignorant one.* The professional speaks a special language which seems an unbreakable code to the layman. He doesn't understand it and it confuses him. A simple lease between a landlord and his tenant, an insurance policy, or a credit agreement with a department store is communicated in legal jargon the ordinary person cannot make sense of. The profession of dentistry is no different.

Some patients have heard the language of dentistry and they may be familiar with a few of the terms like gingivectomy, osteoplasty, and temporomandibular joint. But most are confused by such terms. They have a vague notion of some imposing words, but for the most part they are in the dark. The dental consumer who is in the dark is, consequently, placed in a poor negotiating position. Although you can't get a quickee course in dentistry, a simple working knowledge of basic nomenclature will permit you to ask sensible questions and help you evaluate your dental choices. Let's take the mystery out of "the dontias."

The suffix *dontia* is used to denote a specialty of dentistry, as in ortho*dontia,* the specialty of straightening teeth. There are eight specialties that are recognized by the American Dental Association. The ones you may have heard of are:

> Orthodontia   straightening teeth
> Pedodontia   children's dentistry
> Endodontia   root canal therapy
> Periodontia   diseases of the gums
> Exodontia   oral surgery
> Prosthodontia   artificial tooth replacement

Exactly what do we mean by a specialist? The answer can become rather technical and confusing. Can any dentist just attach a specialist label to himself and hang out a shingle:

> **MARTIN X. SUMMER, D.D.S.**
> **ORTHODONTIST**

Or is the title orthodontist conferred because the dentist has had special training and advanced education? The answer is yes in both cases.

In 36 of the 50 states, a dentist can simply call himself a specialist *by limiting his practice to that particular area.* That means an orthodontist can treat *only* those patients who require straightening of teeth. He can *not* work on other patients; he can *not* fill, extract, or replace teeth. However, it is getting more and more difficult to become a specialist this way. In 14 states, dentists can *not* proclaim a specialty without having first passed a state examination. Those states are: Alaska, Arkansas, Illinois, Kansas, Kentucky, Michigan, Mississippi, Missouri, Nevada, Oklahoma, Oregon, South Carolina, Tennessee, and West Virginia.

The trend is clearly to make it *more* difficult for a dentist to declare himself a specialist. Some feel the application of stringent requirements represents a form of tight union, or "closed shop," to keep competition down. *This means higher fees for you.* Others feel the strict state examinations are necessary to "weed out" incompetent specialists and keep the quality highly monitored. To most patients, unconcerned with that quarrel, the specialist is "the guy who charges more."

To further complicate the question of who is a specialist, the American Dental Association has component societies which confer specialty titles like orthodontist and periodontist on those who have completed additional education in their special area. This usually takes about two years of formal education at the graduate level *beyond the D.D.S.* Dentists who have completed this requirement may then take the test for Board Certification and become Diplomates.

On the other hand, there are many dental groups and societies that confer long and official titles *without* stringent requirements. A dentist may simply apply, pay an initiation fee, and be considered a member of the society. For example, there is the prestigious and select American Association of Endodontics which requires strict qualifying procedures. And there is the American Endodontic Society which confers membership after a quickee one day course in the Sargenti method.* To the layman, the names of both societies are equally imposing. So it's difficult for you, the dental consumer, to know what it is all about. As a general rule, those dentists who are Board Certified are the ones with the greatest amount of extra training. However, Board Certification is no *guarantee* that the specialist is more competent than a non-Board Certified specialist anymore than a Ph.D. professor is a guarantee of a better professor than one with an M.A.

In between all this is a vast meadow of many other societies, groups, and associations that confer membership for various degrees of training. Some memberships may have been earned in a few days; others in several months. Many excellent dentists choose to take intensive week long or month long post graduate courses throughout their careers to update their knowledge. This, of course, is all to their credit. But don't be wowed by every diploma hanging on your dentist's wall.

Whatever the requirements for a specialist may be in your state, it helps to know what each "dontia" means. Let's look at them. What does each one cover? What is their special language? What do they treat? How much do they charge? Let's take the mystery out of "the dontias."

PEDODONTIA

A *pedodontist* is a specialist who restricts his practice to *dentistry for children.*** He is a special brand of dentist trained to be tuned in to

---
*See pp. 159-160.
**In 1973, there were 1225 pedodontists, excluding the Armed Forces.

the psychological and emotional aspects of working with youngsters. He is also especially qualified to treat children with behavioral problems, handicapped children, and children with unusual dental problems. Although most general dentists also do children's dentistry, they may refer the difficult or special child to the pedodontist. Pedodontists have refined their techniques and carefully orchestrated their procedures to deal effectively with these children.

Sometimes the root of the child's behavior problem is the parent. Many times I have heard a parent (or grandparent) threaten, "If you don't behave yourself, I'll call the policeman," or cajole, "If you're good, I'll buy you a present." The use of fear tactics and bribery are the most common parental mistakes. It is no wonder that the dentist confronts a serious problem with such a child. The parent has preconditioned that youngster to expect pain and to be fearful, and no amount of bribes or punishment will erase the terror of a scared child. The pedodontist will adopt a firm but compassionate policy and through his treatment he will be reeducating both the parent and the child.

The field of pedodontia is growing rapidly. In 1963, there were only 100 pedodontists in the United States. Today there are over 1200. Since there are approximately 120,000 dentists, pedodontists represent only 1% of dentists. By comparison, note that there are about 360,000 medical doctors of which 20,000 or about 5% are pediatricians. With one out of 100 dentists limiting to children's dentistry, it is generally necessary to rely on your family dentist for your children's dental work. In fact, depending on the section of the country in which you live, you may find it difficult to locate a pedodontist. If so, don't despair. Many general dentists are capable and tuned in to child psychology. Others may be a poor choice. So although you as an adult may be extremely satisfied with your dentist, don't assume you should take your children to him.

A prominent New Jersey pedodontist has some hints in helping you decide if your dentist is right for your child. "Observe the way he approaches and acts with the child. There are more dentists afraid of children than children afraid of dentists." Ask your dentist straight out if he treats children. Some come right out and say, "I prefer not to." Remember, selecting a dentist for your child is quite independent from selecting a dentist for yourself. There is a different set of guidelines to help you make a wise choice. Consider these:

Are there children's books in the waiting room?
Is there a separate corner for toys or puzzles?
Are there child-size chairs and tables?
Are the dental assistants tuned in to kids or do they treat them like "brats" who are disturbing the office routine?

Be especially observant of your dentist's mannerisms when he is with children. Almost any dog lover can detect another dog lover. A music lover can spot another music lover. Children can sense the dentist who likes them and treats them well. Ask your child if he feels comfortable with your dentist. But ask affirmatively. Don't say, "You're not afraid of Dr. March, are you?" Say, "Dr. March is a good dentist and I really like him. How about you?" A dentist who clearly feels at ease with a child comes across loud and clear. Speak to your neighbors. Find out if they are satisfied with the dentist they use for their children.

If you're paying bills for your children's dental work, you'll want to know what you're paying for. How can you save money and still give your children proper care? It helps if you know something about children's dentistry.

Before Your Baby is Born

Your baby has teeth growing inside his gums *before* he is born. This means the mother can do something about her child's dental health while she's pregnant. Parents want their new babies to have beautiful healthy teeth and gums. They want to prevent their babies from getting a lot of tooth decay. You can start your baby on the road to good teeth by establishing a good, nutritious diet for yourself.

The developing fetus needs calcium, phosphorous, and other nutrients and vitamins to form beautiful teeth. They begin to form as early as the sixth to eighth week of pregnancy. Although you may not see your baby's first tooth until he is six to nine months old, you can begin to help him have healthy teeth *more than a year before that.* Because your baby's developing teeth need nutrients, these must be supplied from the food you are eating every day of your pregnancy. However, contrary to the old misconception, your baby does *not* drain calcium from your own teeth.

Eat well. Give your baby good food to build his developing teeth. Eat a balanced, nutritious diet of meat, proteins, vegetables, fruits, milk, cereals, and bread to supply what your baby needs. Some dentists suggest that a pregnant woman take fluoride vitamins, but it has not been established that fluoride can pass through the placenta to influence the developing teeth. Other dentists feel there is a risk, and fluorides should be given to the baby *only* after his birth. Consult your pediatrician or pedodontist for guidance here.

As for your own teeth, don't neglect them during pregnancy. It is false that a pregnant woman should not go to the dentist. On the contrary, poor dental health on your part can lead to pain, extractions, and other dental problems that can make eating difficult and affect your diet. The best thing you can do for your baby's teeth prenatally, is to eat properly and supply him with the nutrients he needs.

Your own routine dental work can be done while you're pregnant, preferably during the first six months when fewer complications of pregnancy occur. But large scale elective dentistry like multiple crowns is better postponed. Be sure to tell your dentist if you're pregnant so he will *not* take routine X rays. Consult him if you notice puffy, swollen gums which may be the result of a change in your hormone system. He can relieve your symptoms by local cleaning and scaling, and you can follow up with proper home care.

Don't neglect your teeth or your diet. Give your baby a head start!

The First Two Years

Oral gratification is one of your baby's first sensations. From his first cry and his first breath of air, the baby begins to use his mouth. Thereafter, the sucking instinct and the need for food reinforce his need for oral gratification.

There are many questions parents have pertaining to their baby's teeth during the first two years of life.

Which is better, breast feeding or bottle feeding?

One of the earliest decisions you must make is whether to breast or bottle feed your baby. This is a highly personal decision, and you should discuss it with your physician. The method you choose may have an effect on your baby's teeth and jaws. Breast feeding exercises the baby's jaw muscles and influences the development of the dental arches and the position of the teeth.

The prolonged use of some nursing bottles with their artificial nipples may be a contributing factor to the development of crooked teeth in your baby. For example, an artificial nipple with holes that are too large may cause milk to flow from the bottle too rapidly. The baby may develop the habit of thrusting his tongue forward to plug the hole or slow the flow of milk. This can be the onset of a tongue thrusting habit, causing the teeth to shift out of position.

Be careful in selecting the brand of artificial nipples you use. There are nipples on the market that closely duplicate the anatomy of the human breast and nipple, and encourage the baby's jaw muscles to be exercised in the most advantageous way. The Nuk Sauger nipple is highly recommended. Ask your pharmacist to order it especially for you if it is not easily available.

At what age should my baby get his first tooth?

When a baby is born, he usually has no visible teeth. It's an exciting moment when the first tooth appears. The central incisors (front teeth) are generally the first to erupt, somewhere around six months. Usually the lower front teeth erupt before the uppers.

My baby still hasn't any teeth and he's 10 months.

Relax, mother. There is a great deal of latitude in the eruption schedule. It does not indicate in any way that your baby is slow, any more than a baby born with teeth is a genius. By the time your child is two or two-and-one-half years old, all his primary teeth will probably be in place. Remember, there is considerable latitude.

What can I do to help my baby while he's teething?

Teething is a natural process. It is not an illness. Little bumps appear on the gums that are the outline of the teeth fighting to break through. Some people believe you should take the infant to the dentist and have him lance the gums to help the teeth cut through faster.

This is nonsense. Since teething is a natural process, Mother Nature will arrange the schedule. Your baby may exhibit signs of drooling and discomfort during teething along with crying and fretfulness, but illness accompanied by fever is not normal during teething. If your child is ill, call your physician. He may suggest aspirin or Tylenol drops. Numbing agents are only temporary and may sensitize your baby to benzocaine.

How important are baby teeth?

Your baby's primary teeth are necessary for eating, speaking, facial growth, and appearance. They act as a guide to help the permanent teeth erupt into their proper places. These teeth should be provided with all necessary care and treatment until they are lost. Premature loss of primary teeth due to neglect can cause considerable problems to permanent teeth. Don't let anyone talk you into neglecting baby teeth because "they aren't important and they fall out anyhow." This short sighted and erroneous idea will hurt your baby. You won't save money, and you could wind up spending a lot on orthodontic treatments to straighten your child's teeth later on.

When should I start and stop fluoride treatments?

Ideally, your child should receive fluorides in the community drinking water from birth on. This will help develop decay resistant teeth.

If your water supply is not fluoridated, by all means ask your dentist about alternate methods of fluoridation. Even if your community water supply does contain fluoride, it is a good idea to supplement this with topical fluoride treatments and fluoride vitamins. Fluorides are effective only on develop*ING* teeth, and do not have a beneficial effect on develop*ED* teeth.

Fluoride treatments should be applied regularly from age two (once every 6-12 months) until all your child's permanent teeth have erupted. The proper application of topical fluoride treatments coupled with ingesting fluorides from community water can reduce tooth decay *as much as 65%*. So if you have reduced decay, you have also reduced your child's dental bills. A wise dental consumer will see that his children receive adequate fluoride protection.

The following cities have fluoride in their drinking water

Alabama
Albertville
Anniston
Athens
Auburn
Boaz
Dothan
Fairfax
Fayette
Florence
Ft. Payne
Geraldine
Gordo
Henagar
Holt
Huntsville
Jacksonville
Lafayette
Langdale
Livingston
Mobile
Montevallo
Northport
Oneonta
Oxford
Rainsville
River View
Russellville
Section
Shawmut
Sheffield
Sylvania
Tuscaloosa
Tuscumbia
York

Alaska
Anchorage
Douglas
Sitka

Arkansas
Alexander
Arkadelphia
Batesville
Benton
Bentonville
Clarksville
Conway
Crossett
Dumas
Eden Isle
Forrest City
Harrison
Helena
Hope
Jacksonville
Jonesboro
Judsonia
Lewisville
Little Rock
Mabelvale
Madison
Marianna
Morrilton
Newport
Osceola
Paragould
Prescott
Russellville
Searcy
Springdale
Star City
Sweet Home
Waldo
Warren
West Helena
West Memphis
Wrightsville
Yellville

California
Antioch
Avenal
Baywood Park
Broadmoor
Burlingame
Colma
Concord
Gridley
Hayward
Hillsborough
Los Banos
Martinez
Mount View
Oroville
Pacifica
Palo Alto
Pittsburg
Placerville
Pleasanton
Port Chicago
Rosemont
Roseville
San Bruno
San Carlos
San Francisco
San Luis Obispo
San Mateo
Vallejo

Colorado
Aurora
Berthoud
Craig
Denver
Durango
Edgewater
Grand Junction
Greeley
Lafayette
Lakewood
Longmont
Loveland
Monte Vista
Montrose
Palisade
Sheridan
Timnath
Wheat Ridge
Windsor

Connecticut
Berlin
Bloomfield
Bristol
Cromwell
Glastonbury
Hartford
Middletown
New Britain
New Canaan
Newington
Stonington
Torrington
West Mystic
Wethersfield
Willimantic
Windsor

Delaware
Lewes
Newark
Selbyville
Wilmington

District of Columbia
Washington, D.C.

Florida
Bal Harbour
Belle Glade
Clewiston
Cocoa Beach
Coral Gables
Ft. Pierce
Gainesville
Hialeah
Kendall
Key West
Miami
Miami Beach
Naples
Ocala
Orlando
Rockledge

Georgia
Acworth
Albany
Athens
Augusta
Austell
Baldwin
Barnesville
Bogart
Buford
Calhoun
Canton
Cartersville
Chamblee
Clarkdale
Cornelia
Covington
Decatur
Doraville
Dublin
East Griffin
Eastman
Elberton
Experiment
Fairburn
Fairview
Fitzgerald
Forsyth
Ft. Valley
Gainesville
Garden Lakes
Griffin
Hogansville
Holly Springs
Kennesaw
Lafayette
Manchester
Marietta
Montezuma
Monticello
Newnan
North Canton
Oxford
Pine Lake
Plainville
Princeton
Rome
Rossville
Smyrna
Statesboro
Thomaston
Thomasville
Valdosta
Warner Robins
West Point
Winterville

Hawaii
Maunaloa

Idaho
Bonners Ferry
Council
Jerome
Kootenai
Lewiston
McCall
Meridian
Montepelier
Orofino
Ponderay
Preston
Salmon
Sand point
Shoshone

Illinois
Alsip
Amboy
Assumption
Bannockburn
Beckemeyer
Bedford Park
Bellevue
Berwyn
Blue Island
Bluford
Bradley
Bridgeport
Brookfield
Calumet City
Calumet Park
Carbondale
Casey
Catlin
Charleston
Chester
Chicago
Cicero
Colp
Dalton City
Danville
Decatur
Deerfield
Dolton
Du Quoin
Effingham
Elmwood Park
Energy
Eureka
Evanston
Forest Park
Franklin Park
Galesburg
Glencoe
Glenview
Harvey
Hazelcrest
Herrin
Highland Park
Hillside

Hodgkins
Hometown
Jerseyville
Kankakee
Kenilworth
La Grange
La Salle
Lake Forest
Lanark
Lansing
Lebanon
Lincolnwood
Lyons
Marion
Matteson
Maywood
McCook
Melrose Park
Midlothian
Moline
Morton Grove
Mt. Vernon
Mt. Zion
Murphysboro
Newton
Niles
Normal
Northbrook
Northfield
Oak Lawn
Oak Park
Orion
Park Forest
Peoria
Phoenix
Pittsfield
Posen
Quincy
Rankin
River Forest
River Grove
Riverside
Robinson
Rock Island
Rosemont
Rosiclare
St. Johns
Salem
Sesser
Skokie
Sparta
Steelville
Stone Park
Sullivan
Summit
Sumner
Taylorville
Valier
Vergennes
Waukegan
Westchester
Wheaton

Wheeling
White Hall
Wilmette
Winnetka

Indiana

Algiers
Anderson
Batesville
Bedford
Black Oak
Bloomfield
Brazil
Carmel
Coalmont
Columbus
Corydon
Culver
Dale
Edgewood
Elkhart
Evansville
Fortville
Ft. Wayne
Gary
Greendale
Greensburg
Griffith
Hammond
Harmony
Highland
Huntingburg
Indianapolis
Jasonville
Jasper
Kokomo
Lafayette
La Porte
Logansport
Long Beach
Lyndhurst
Marion
Martinsville
Maywood
Michigan City
Mishawaka
Montgomery
Montpelier
Mt. Vernon
Muncie
New Carlisle
New Castle
North Vernon
Oldenburg
Paoli
Princeton
Rensselaer
Richmond
Rushville
Seymour
Southport
Valparaiso

Vevay
Wabash
Walkerton
Waynedale
Winamac
Zionsville

Iowa

Ames
Audubon
Avoca
Bancroft
Belmond
Bettendorf
Boone
Burlington
Carlisle
Cedar Falls
Cedar Rapids
Centerville
Chariton
Clarinda
Clinton
Clive
Corning
Council Bluffs
Cresco
Creston
Davenport
Decorah
Des Moines
Eagle Grove
Eldora
Emmetsburg
Fairfield
Glenwood
Greenfield
Hartley
Humboldt
Iowa City
Jefferson
Keokuk
Lake View
Lamoni
Manchester
Marion
Monticello
Newton
Oskaloosa
Ottumwa
Perry
Postville
Red Oak
Sac City
St. Ansgar
Sigourney
Sioux Center
Sioux Rapids
Tipton
Urbandale
Waukon
Winterset

Kansas

Arkansas City
Ashland
Bonner Springs
Burlington
Chanute
Clearwater
Coffeyville
Council Grove
Edwardsville
El Dorado
Emporia
Eureka
Fairway
Ft. Scott
Fredonia
Hays
Herington
Independence
Kansas City
La Harpe
Lawrence
Lyons
Marion
Olathe
Ottawa
Paola
Parsons
Phillipsburg
Seneca
Shawnee
Stafford
Topeka
Yates Center

Kentucky

Aflex
Anchorage
Ashland
Bardstown
Bardwell
Beattyville
Bellewood
Benton
Berea
Broad Fields
Buechel
Burgin
Burkesville
Calvert City
Cambridge
Carrollton
Central City
Cherry Wood
Cynthiana
Danville
Devondale
Druid Hills
Elkton
Eminence
Fairmeade
Frankfort

Franklin
Glasgow
Graymoor
Grayson
Greensburg
Hardinsburg
Harrodsburg
Hazard
Henderson
Hickman
Hopkinsville
Hustonville
Irvine
Jackson
Jett
Junction City
Kingsley
La Grange
Lancer
Lebanon
Lexington
Louisa
Louisville
Lynch
Lyndon
Lynnview
Martin
Mayfield
Maysville
Middletown
Mockingbird
Morehead
Morgantown
Mt. Sterling
Murray
New Castle
Owensboro
Paintsville
Paris
Pikeville
Prestonsburg
Richlawn
Russellville
St. Matthews
Scottsville
Shelbyville
Shively
Springfield
Springlee
Sturgis
Taylorsville
Thealka
Vanceburg
Versailles
Wellington
Winchester

Louisiana

Houma
Jonesville
Lockport
Rayville
Thibodaux

TAKING THE MYSTERY OUT OF "THE DONTIAS"   135

Maine
Baileyville
Bar Harbor
Belfast
Bradley
Bridgton
Brunswick
Caribou
Fairfield
Hampden
Jackman
Madawaska
Milford
Millinocket
Mount Desert
Norway
Old Town
Pittsfield
Presque Isle
Rumford
Topsham
Vassalboro
Veazie
Waterville
Winslow

Maryland
Aberdeen
Adelphi
Alta Vista
Anapolis
Anneslie
Arbutus
Ardwick
Avalon
Baltimore
Bare Hills
Baynesville
Bel Air
Beltsville
Berwyn
Bladensburg
Brentwood
Cabin John
Carney
Catonsville
Cavetown
Chesaco Park
Cheverly
Chevy Chase
Cockeysville
College Park
Colmar Manor
Cottage City
Dumbarton
Dundalk
Eastport
Edgemere
Edmonston
Elkridge
Essex
Fairtown

Fitzell
Forest Glen
Forestville
Four Corners
Frederick
Fullerton
Funkstown
Gaithersburg
Garrett Park
Glen Echo
Glen Mont
Glyndon
Golden Ring
Greenbelt
Hagerstown
Halethorpe
Harbor View
Harristown
Hebbville
Hillendale
Hyattsville
Idlewild
Inverness
Kensington
Kenwood
Landover
Lanham
Lansdowne
Larchmont
Laurel
Lenox
Linhigh
Loch Raven
Lodge Forest
Lutherville
Middle River
Milford
Monumental
Morningside
Mt. Rainier
Necker
North East
North Point
Oak Forest
Overlea
Padonia
Paradise
Parkville
Perry Hall
Pikesville
Pinehurst
Ralston
Riderwood
Riggs Road
Riverdale
River Neck
Rockdale
Rockland
Rockville
Rosedale
Rosemont
Roslyn

Rossville
Ruxton
Salisbury
Seabrook
Security
Sheppard
Silver Hill
Silver Spring
Smithsburg
Snow Hill
Stemmers Run
Stoneleigh
Suitland
Takoma Park
Texas
Timonium
Towson
Turner
Villa Nova
Walters
West Gate
Westminster
Wheaton
Williamsport
Woodbrook
Woodside

Massachusetts
Ashburnham
Athol
Beverly
Cohasset
Danvers
Hamilton
Hingham
Hull
Middleton
Newton
Salem
Seekonk
Sharon
Shrewsbury
Sudbury
Templeton
Winchester

Michigan
Adrian
Algonac
Ann Arbor
Battle Creek
Bayview
Benton Harbor
Big Rapids
Brighton
Buchanan
Center Line
Central Lake
Charlevoix
Charlotte
Chelsea
East Jordan
East Lansing

Escanaba
Essexville
Frankenmuth
Gladstone
Grand Haven
Grand Rapids
Grandville
Hastings
Hillsdale
Howell
Jackson
Kalamazoo
Lansing
Lowell
Ludington
Manistique
Marine City
Marion
Marquette
Marysville
Mason
Menominee
Midland
Milford
Monroe
Mt. Clemens
Muskegon
Negaunee
Parchment
Pearl Beach
Petoskey
Pinconning
Plainwell
Rockford
Rogers City
Sheridan
South Haven
Sparta
Spring Lake
Stambaugh
Tecumseh
West Branch
White Pine
Wyoming
Yale
Ypsilanti

Minnesota
Albert Lea
Anoka
Arlington
Askov
Aurora
Bayport
Benson
Bird Island
Blaine
Bloomington
Blue Earth
Buffalo
Cloquet
Crookston
Crystal

Dassel
Edgerton
Edina
Excelsior
Fergus Falls
Foley
Forest Lake
Gaylord
Hallock
Hopkins
Hoyt Lakes
Hutchinson
Lakefield
Litchfield
Madison
Mankato
Marshall
Minneapolis
Montevideo
Moorhead
Morningside
Morris
Northfield
Olivia
Ortonville
Perham
Pine Island
Pipestone
Ranier
Richfield
Robbinsdale
Rochester
Roseville
Rush City
Sauk Centre
Scanlon
Silver Bay
Springfield
Staples
Truman
Virginia
Waterville
Wayzata
West Concord
Windom
Winnebago
Winona

Mississippi
Brookhaven
Calhoun City
Canton
Cleveland
Columbia
Columbus
Como
Durant
Forest
Kosciusko
Lexington
Louisville
Marks
Meridian

136 HOW TO SAVE YOUR TEETH AND YOUR MONEY

Newton
Philadelphia
Quitman
Tupelo
Union
Missouri
Albany
Ballwin
Berkeley
Bevier
Boonville
Brentwood
Bridgeton
Brookfield
Cabool
Cameron
Cape Girardeau
Carthage
Chaffee
Champ
Charlack
Chillicothe
Clayton
Clinton
Cool Valley
Crestwood
Creve Coeur
Crystal City
Dellwood
Des Peres
Edmundson
Ellisville
Elmdale
Fenton
Ferguson
Festus
Florissant
Frontenac
Gilliam
Glasgow
Glendale
Greendale
Hanley Hills
Hannibal
Hayti
Hazelwood
Hillhouse
Jackson
Jefferson City
Jennings
Kennett
Kirkwood
La Due
Lakeshire
Lamar
Liberty
Mackenzie
Macon
Manchester
Marceline
Marlborough

Mary Ridge
Maryville
Moline Acres
Normandy
Oakland
Overland
Pacific
Pagedale
Perryville
Pine Lawn
Plattsburg
Richland
Riverview
Rock Hill
Salisbury
Sarcoxie
Savannah
Shelbina
Shrewsbury
Sikeston
Slater
Sunset Hills
Times Beach
Twin Oaks
Unionville
Uplands Park
Valley Park
Versailles
Vinita Park
Warson Woods
Wellston
Wilbur Park
Winchester
Montana
Bozeman
Conrad
Miles City
Roundup
St. Ignatius
Nebraska
Columbus
Fairbury
Nebraska City
Superior
Nevada
Owyhee
New Hampshire
Durham
Hanover
Lebanon
New Jersey
Allenhurst
Atlantic City
Burlington
Deal
E. Brunswick
Eatontown
Fair Haven
Far Hills
Highland Park

Interlaken
Little Silver
Long Branch
Middletown
Neptune City
Ocean Grove
Ocean Port
Perth Amboy
Princeton
Rahway
Roosevelt
Rumson
Sea Bright
Trenton
Wharton
Woodbridge
New Mexico
Abiquiu
Agua Fria
Anton Chico
Capulin
Cordova
Cundiyo
East Pecos
Glorieta
La Placita
Penasco
Raton
Rio Lucio
Ruidoso
Santa Fe
Sena
Taos
Vadito
Valdez
Valley Ranch
Wagon Mound
New York
Allegany
Ardsley
Batavia
Belfast
Binghamton
Bronxville
Buffalo
Canandaigua
Castile
Celoron
Chenango
Cobleskill
Delhi
Dickinson
Dobbs Ferry
Dresden
East Aurora
Eastchester
Elmira
Elmsford
Fairport
Falconer
Geneseo

Gloversville
Greece
Greenburgh
Hamburg
Hastings
Highland
Hilton
Honeoye Falls
Hoosick Falls
Hopewell
Hudson Falls
Jamestown
Johnstown
Kenmore
Lakewood
Larchmont
Levittown
Lewiston
Livonia
Lloyd
Lockport
Macedon
Mamaroneck
Medina
Middleport
Mineola
Monticello
Mount Vernon
New Rochelle
New York City
Newark
Newburgh
Newfane
Niagara Falls
Niskayuna
Ogden
Olean
Oneonta
Oswego
Palmyra
Parmatown
Pelham
Pelham Manor
Penfield
Penn Yan
Perinton
Perry
Phelps
Pittsford
Plattsburgh
Porter
Poughkeepsie
Rochester
Rotterdam
Saranac Lake
Scarsdale
Schenectady
Scriba
Syracuse
Tonawanda
Tuckahoe
Vestal

Walden
Warsaw
Watertown
Webster
Westfield
Wheatfield
Yonkers
North Carolina
Aberdeen
Albemarle
Brookford
Carrboro
Chapel Hill
Charlotte
Concord
Dallas
Dunn
Durham
East Spencer
Eden
Erwin
Fayetteville
Gastonia
Goldsboro
Greenville
Hickory
High Point
Laurinburg
Lenoir
Lexington
Lillington
Longhurst
Lowell
Lumberton
Misenheimer
Monroe
Morganton
Mount Airy
New Bern
New London
Newton
Pineville
Raleigh
Ranlo
Reidsville
Richfield
Rockingham
Rocky Mount
Roxboro
Ruth
Salisbury
Sanford
Shelby
Smithfield
Spindale
Statesville
Tarboro
Washington
Wilmington
Wilson

TAKING THE MYSTERY OUT OF "THE DONTIAS"   137

North Dakota
Belcourt
Beulah
Bismarck
Carrington
Cavalier
Crosby
Devils Lake
Dickinson
Drayton
Fargo
Grand Forks
Jamestown
Mandan
Minot
Riverdale
Rugby
Valley City
Walhalla
Williston

Ohio
Amherst
Avon
Avon Lake
Bay Village
Beachwood
Bedford
Berea
Brecksville
Brook Park
Brooklyn
Canfield
Chesapeake
Cleveland
Coal Grove
Eastlake
Elyria
Euclid
Findlay
Gallipolis
Gate Mills
Georgetown
Girard
Glendale
Hamilton
Harbor View
Harrisville
Haskins
Holland
Hudson
Huron
Independence
Ironton
Jackson
Lakeline
Lakewood
Lisbon
Lorain
Lyndhurst
Madeira
Marietta

Maumee
Mayfield
McDonald
Medina
New Boston
Newark
Niles
Northfield
Oberlin
Orange
Oregon
Orrville
Ottawa Hills
Parkview
Parma
Pepper Pike
Perrysburg
Portsmouth
Rocky River
Rossford
Salem
Shaker Heights
Sheffield
Solon
South Euclid
Strongsville
Terrace Park
Timberlake
Toledo
Tontogany
Vermilion
Wadsworth
Walton Hills
Waterville
West View
Westerville
Wickliffe
Willoughby
Yellow Springs
Youngstown

Oklahoma
Ada
Altus
Atoka
Bartlesville
Clinton
Dewey
Guthrie
Hydro
Idabel
McAlester
Midwest City
Norman
Nowata
Oklahoma City
Pawhuska
Ponca City
Shawnee
Stillwater
Tulsa

Oregon
Astoria
Cedar Hills
Charleston
Coos Bay
Coquille
Dallas
East Salem
Eastside
Florence
Forest Grove
Gearhart
Gold Beach
Hammond
McMinnville
Mill City
Newport
North Bend
Pendleton
Salem
Sublimity
Sweet Home
Turner
Warm Springs
Warrenton

Pennsylvania
Arnold
Baldwin
Bedford
Bethel
Brackenridge
Braddock
Brentwood
Bridgeville
Bridgewater
Brookville
Burgettstown
Camp Hill
Carlisle
Carnegie
Catasauqua
Chalfont
Chambersburg
Chester Hill
Churchill
Clarion
Crafton
Cumberland
Dormont
Du Bois
Easton
Ebensburg
Finleyville
Ford City
Forest Hills
Greentree
Greenville
Harrison
Heidelberg
Homestead
Indiana

Ingram
Jefferson
Kane
Kittanning
Lancaster
Lemoyne
Library
Manheim
Manor
Manorville
Mansfield
McDonald
Media
Millersburg
Mt. Oliver
Munhall
Natrona
New Castle
North East
Osborne
Patton
Perryopolis
Philadelphia
Philipsburg
Pitcairn
Pittsburgh
Quarryville
Ridgway
Scott
Sewickley
Sharpsville
Shenango
Shiremanstown
Somerset
State College
Swissvale
Thornburg
Trafford
Turtle Creek
Uniontown
West Homestead
West Mifflin
Whitehall
Wilkinsburg
Williams
Wilmerding
Wilson
Wormleysburg

Rhode Island
Barrington
Bristol
Cranston
Johnston
Middletown
Newport
Pawtucket
Portsmouth
Providence
Smithfield
Warren
Warwick

Woonsocket

South Carolina
Aiken
Bishopville
Cheraw
Chester
Chesterfield
Clemson
Clinton
Darlington
Fort Mill
Hartsville
Honea Path
Johnston
Lancaster
Marion
Ninety Six
No. Augusta
Orangeburg
Rock Hill
Seneca
Summerville
Sumter
Union
Westminster
Winnsboro
York

South Dakota
Aberdeen
Brookings
Hosmer
Huron
Mitchell
Mobridge
Vermillion
Watertown

Tennessee
Alamo
Alcoa
Arlington
Athens
Bartlett
Bristol
Brownsville
Chapel Hill
Chattanooga
Clarksville
Cleveland
Clifton
Columbia
Cookeville
Covington
Cowan
Decatur
Decherd
Dresden
Dunlap
Dyersburg
East Ridge
Erwin

Ethridge
Fayetteville
Flat Woods
Franklin
Gallatin
Germantown
Harriman
Hartsville
Hixson
Humboldt
Jackson
Johnson City
Kingsport
La Follette
Lakewood
La Vergne
Lebanon
Linden
Livingston
Manchester
Maryville
Milan
Millington
Mt. Pleasant
Nashville
Newport
Niota
Oak Ridge
Paris
Parsons
Perryville
Pikeville
Portland
Raleigh
Ridgely
Ripley
Savannah
Sewanee
Shelbyville
Smyrna
So. Bristol
Sparta
Springfield
Tiptonville
Trenton
Union City
Waverly
Waynesboro
Winchester
Woodbine
Woodbury

Texas

Breckenridge
Center
Conroe
Crockett
Denton
Fort Worth
Gonzales
Gregory
Griffing Park

Ingleside
Iowa Park
Killeen
Lakeview
Lawrence
Marshall
Mesquite
Muenster
Odem
Paris
Pear Ridge
Port Arthur
Portland
Sabine Pass
Sweetwater
Temple
Terrell
Trent
Wellington

Utah

Helper

Vermont

Burlington
Derby Line
Essex Junction
Swanton

Virginia

Alexandria
Amherst
Annandale
Bedford
Blacksburg
Bluefield
Bristol
Charlottesville
Chatham
Chesapeake
Danville
Dublin
Dumfries
Fairfax
Falls Church
Falmouth
Farmville
Fredericksburg
Front Royal
Fries
Hampton
Harrisonburg
Lakeside
Lexington
Lynchburg
Newport News
Norfolk
Norton
Petersburg
Portsmouth
Pulaski
Radford
Richmond

Roanoke
Rocky Mount
Springfield
Staunton
Suffolk
Vinton
Virginia Beach
Warrenton
Waynesboro
Wise
Woodbridge
Wytheville
Yorktown

Washington

Anacortes
Cathlamet
Centralia
Coulee Dam
Duvall
Forks
Kalama
Kelso
Kent
Kirkland
Longview
Lynden
Manson
Montesano
Oak Harbor
Pullman
Raymond
Vancouver
Woodland

West Virginia

Alpheus
Anmoore
Beckley
Benton Ferry
Benwood
Bethlehem
Bridgeport
Buckhannon
Burke Hollow
Cameron
Charleston
Chesapeake
Chester
Clarksburg
Clearview
Colfax
Cross Lanes
Dakota
Diamond
Dunbar
Elbert
Elkins
Fairmont
Fairview
Fayetteville
Filbert
Glen Jean

Glenville
Grafton
Grantsville
Harrisville
Harvey
Henderson
Hugheston
Huntington
Hurricane
Institute
Jane Lew
Kingmont
Kingwood
Lens Creek
Lewisburg
Lochgelly
Logan
London
Man
Martinsburg
Matewan
McConnell
Milton
Montgomery
Morgantown
Mt. Gay
Nitro
North Fork
Oak Hill
Parkview
Peach Creek
Philippi
Pinch
Pineville
Poca
Princeton
Quincy
Rand
Red Jacket
Ripley
Rivesville
Rowlesburg
Shrewsbury
Sistersville
Spring Hill
Stollings
Summerlee
Summersville
Sun Valley
Terra Alta
Thorpe
Triadelphia
Union
Vienna
Wayne
Weirton
Welch
Wellsburg
Wheatland
Wheeling
Whipple
Wilcoe

Williamson
Williamstown
Winfield
Winifrede

Wisconsin

Albany
Alma
Amery
Argyle
Ashland
Baraboo
Beaver Dam
Belleville
Beloit
Benton
Berlin
Black Earth
Blair
Blue River
Boscobel
Brodhead
Brooklyn
Burke
Caledonia
Cambridge
Cassville
Cedarburg
Clinton
Cobb
Coloma
Columbus
Cuba City
Darlington
De Forest
Dickeyville
Durand
East Troy
Eau Claire
Edgar
Edgerton
Elkhorn
Evansville
Fall River
Fennimore
Fond Du Lac
Footville
Fox Point
Frederic
Friesland
Galesville
Glendale
Grantsburg
Green Bay
Greendale
Greenfield
Hartford
Hayward
Hazel Green
Hudson
Janesville
Jefferson

Kenosha	Milwaukee	Osceola	Saint Francis	Wausau
Keshena	Mondovi	Oshkosh	Sheboygan	Wauwatosa
Kohler	Monona	Pardeeville	Shell Lake	West Allis
Lake Geneva	Monticello	Park Falls	Shorewood	West Baraboo
Lake Mills	Mosinee	Pewaukee	Shullsburg	West Bend
Lancaster	Mount Horeb	Plain	Sparta	Weyauwega
Lodi	Mukwonago	Platteville	Spooner	Whitehall
Livingston	Muscoda	Port Edwards	Spring Green	Williams Bay
Madison	Neillsville	Portage	Stoughton	Windsor
Maple Bluff	Nekoosa	Potosi	Sturgeon Bay	Wonewoc
Marinette	Neopit	Poynette	Sun Prairie	**Wyoming**
Mayville	New Glarus	Racine	Tennyson	
Mazomanie	New Holstein	Reedsburg	Tomahawk	Laramie
McFarland	New Richmond	Rice Lake	Trempealeau	Saratoga
Menasha	North Hudson	Rio	Two Rivers	Sinclair
Merrill	Oconomowoc	Ripon	Waterloo	Thermopolis
Middleton	Omro	River Falls	Watertown	
Milton	Oregon	Rothschild	Waunakee	

*Partial Listing.

In the future, there may be over-the-counter, non-prescription fluoride gels and fluoride rinses available for home use.

Your baby is a thumb sucker.

Thumb sucking, during the early years, is a normal instinct. It provides a feeling of security and pleasure to the baby. During the first few years, thumb sucking is no cause for alarm. Usually, a child will taper off this habit and perhaps suck only at night to fall asleep. If thumb or finger sucking persists past the age of seven, it can cause a shifting of the permanent teeth and a malocclusion can develop. Parents and dentists alike have tried scores of habit breaking devices.
One of these is a "hay rake," an appliance made and cemented into place by the dentist, containing sharp barbs to discourage the finger from being placed in the mouth. Another method is to paint foul smelling and tasting solutions on the child's fingers. Attempts to break the habit range from outright punishment, to elaborate splints placed over the child's finger. Often, the method is more damaging than the habit. A psychiatrist summed up his assessment of the problem saying, "A malocclusion of the mind is more serious than a malocclusion of the mouth."
Parents often use pacifiers to satisfy their baby's sucking instinct and to discourage thumb sucking. If you buy a pacifier, be sure it is

not easily swallowed or broken. In March 1976, *The New York Times* reported the roundup of 50,000 baby pacifiers in the New York, New Jersey area after the death of a five month old Bronx infant from asphyxiation. Over 150,000 pacifiers imported to the United States from Spain under the names Fauna, Hermetic, Texas, and Navy were recalled by the United States Food and Drug Administration for potential choking and aspiration hazards to infants. Watch out for dangerous teething rings, too: those filled with liquid containing ammonia which can cause vomiting or bacterial contamination. Some trade under the names Protecto Gum Soother, Protecto Cool Ring Gum Soother, Baby World Teether, and Charm Fun Candy Pacifiers. If you buy your baby a pacifier, make sure the shield is not so flexible or so small that it can easily be swallowed.

Your child is a tongue thruster.

Some children develop a habit of pressing their tongue forward against the teeth when swallowing. This phenomenon is called "tongue thrusting" or "reverse swallowing," and may have developed from using an artificial nipple with too large a hole. This habit can cause crooked teeth. The pressure exerted by the tongue pressing against the teeth has enough force to move teeth out of their proper position. Ask your pedodontist about this. He may refer you to an orthodontist or suggest myofunctional therapy (reeducation and special exercises involved in the swallowing pattern).

Your child is only two and has developed many cavities.

Yes, a child of two can have lots of cavities. This is called Nursing Bottle Mouth. It occurs when a baby is allowed to fall asleep in his crib or carriage with the bottle "propped" in his mouth. A baby should be held and cuddled while being fed. If the baby is not held and the bottle is propped with a pillow, the baby may fall asleep with the bottle fluids still in his mouth. The warmth of the mouth plus certain bacteria in the mouth change the sugar to decay-causing acid, forming a perfect medium for the decay process. Restoration and filling of multiple cavities on a two year old can be extremely difficult or impossible, and your child can lose valuable teeth.

> **Warning: Bottle Propping Costs Money**
>
> *Do not prop the bottle and allow milk or sweetened drinks to lodge around your baby's teeth while he sleeps. This can cause great harm and cost you hundreds of dollars in dental bills.*

At what age should you start brushing your child's teeth?

You can start to brush your baby's teeth shortly after the first teeth appear. A wet toothbrush without toothpaste can be the starter. Make a game of it. Of course, parental supervision will be necessary for a few years, but many preschoolers like to imitate their parents and they will take over by themselves. Be sure to buy them a toothbrush that is small enough and try to make it a pleasurable experience. Make sure you give them toothpaste with fluoride.

At what age should I take my child for his first dental visit?

Your child should visit the dentist no later than two or two-and-one-half. The first visit should simply be a "get acquainted visit," and this introduction should be as pleasant as possible. Surveys show that 50% of two year olds have one or more decayed teeth. The first dental visit should be made before your child develops a toothache. Unfortunately, countless thousands of children are brought to the dentist for the first time with an aching tooth. They arrive at the office screaming in pain, fear, and terror. This set of circumstances helps perpetuate the myth that dentistry is painful, and dental visits thereafter are associated with pain. Don't indoctrinate your child with this sort of dental experience. These are the children who grow up fearing the dentist and avoiding dental treatment.

Six to Twelve Years

This period is marked by the appearance of the first permanent molar, called "the six year molar." Also, by the age of six, the roots of the baby teeth are beginning to resorb and the permanent teeth start to make their way to the surface. It is also during this period that all the permanent teeth usually appear in the mouth (except wisdom teeth). Here are the most common questions parents want to know about their 6-12 year olds.

At what age do the permanent teeth come in?

The first permanent molar usually erupts around age six. This tooth is a key tooth in the mouth, and should be preserved and maintained for the balance of life. There may be some discomfort in cutting this molar, and it should not be confused with a sore throat. The six year molar does not replace a baby tooth. Neither does the 12 year molar or wisdom tooth. The jaw accommodates these additions. Remember, there are 20 baby teeth and 32 permanent teeth. Don't confuse the six year molar with a baby tooth. It is a pivotal tooth in the developing jaw and should not be neglected.

My child is ten years old, how long should I continue these fluoride treatments?

Under optimum circumstances, topical fluorides should continue at least until all the permanent teeth have erupted (excluding wisdom teeth). In this way, every permanent tooth will have the opportunity to receive the benefits of fluoride. Continue to have your child use fluoride toothpaste. This, too, will reduce cavities.

Should a baby tooth be extracted if it is causing a toothache?

Your six year old has been up all night with a toothache. Your dentist explains that the baby tooth is infected and is the cause of the pain. His X ray indicates that the replacement tooth still has another 3-4 years before it erupts. Even though the offending tooth is only a baby tooth, he advises you to save it with a routine procedure called "a pulpotomy." This is somewhat similar to root canal therapy, but simpler and much less costly.

A pedodontist can perform a pulpotomy* in one visit and the tooth could then remain pain free to guide the permanent tooth into place. All this can be accomplished for a fee of about $40. On the

---

*Removal of the upper portion of the pulp (nerve).

other hand, if the tooth is extracted and not replaced, adjacent teeth can drift into the extraction space, causing thousands of dollars of orthodontic bills. It makes good consumer economics to spend $40 to avoid a possible $1500 bill later on.

Warning: Not all dentists can or will perform a pulpotomy on a child who, in all probability, has been up all night in pain. The screaming is upsetting to other patients in the waiting rooms, is throwing the dentist off schedule (he worked you in on an emergency basis), and he may not be willing or able to cope with a distressed parent and a frantic child. It's far easier for him to extract the baby tooth than spend time explaining what a pulpotomy is to a skeptical parent whose reaction might be, "What? $40 to fix a baby tooth?" Even if he can convince the parent, he must then face up to performing the work under difficult circumstances — another half hour of demanding and tiring work. *Don't be talked into an extraction under these circumstances, although it might appear to be the easy way out.* A wise dental consumer will question his dentist about a pulpotomy to save the tooth. The baby tooth is a *natural* space maintainer. A toothache in a baby tooth does *not* mean the tooth should be extracted.

What is a space maintainer?

A space maintainer is an artificial device that prevents adjacent teeth from drifting into a space created by the extraction of a baby tooth. It might cost about $50. If a baby tooth has been lost prematurely, then a space maintainer is indicated. Like a pulpotomy, it can save you thousands of dollars in future orthodontic bills. Don't overlook this simple and effective method of saving money. As a general rule, the pulpotomy is preferable. The space maintainer is called for when an extraction of a baby tooth is unavoidable.

Teenage Dentistry

By the age of 13, all the permanent teeth, with the exception of the wisdom teeth, have erupted. Your child is starting to leave the pedodontic stage of dentistry and is beginning to be treated as an adult. It is during this teenage period that most young people experience the most decay. Hormonal changes, rapid growth spurts, erratic eating habits, consumption of junk foods, and poor oral hygiene contribute to the high rate of decay.

Junk Food Junkies

The State Board of Education in West Virginia voted to remove all candy, soda, gum, and flavored ice bars from the kids' school vending machines. Empty machines? Not at all. They've replaced them with yogurt, soup, fruit, and juices. What spurred this sharp action? A survey showed the school kids were turning into "junk-food-junkies."

For these reasons, it is imperative that frequent dental checkups be backed up with scrupulous oral hygiene. At no other time in life is physical appearance a greater measure of popularity and success than during the teenage years. The teenager is now becoming interested in his own mouth and especially in the appearance of his teeth and smile. He is now entering the orthodontic years.

Teenagers with permanent teeth should start to become wise dental consumers, too. Words like orthodontia, root canal, and gingivitis, should become part of their vocabulary. Each new generation should become more informed than the last. A wise dental consumer can begin as a teenager.

Teen Teeth Troubles

The average 16 year old American teenager has 10 decayed teeth that are untreated. Sound terrible? In England it's even worse. The twenty-first birthday present for many Yorkshire lads and lassies is a full set of dentures. In Great Britain, one out of three people over 16 have NO natural teeth.

PEDODONTIC CONSUMER TIPS

- Be sure to tell your dentist if you are pregnant, so he does not take X rays. This can be dangerous to your baby.
- Don't miss your own dental appointments when you're pregnant.
- Give your children fluorides to reduce decay up to 65%.
- Don't use bottle nipples with large holes. You may be encouraging tongue thrusting, which can cost you high orthodontic or myofunctional bills.
- Don't prop your baby's bottle. The milk or juice lodged around the teeth can contribute to rampant decay and large dental bills.
- Take your child to the dentist by age two to two-and-a-half, *before* he has a toothache.
- A $40 pulpotomy can preserve a baby tooth and save you $1500 in orthodontic fees. Don't have a baby tooth extracted because it hurts.
- If a baby tooth is prematurely lost, ask about a space maintainer to save the space for the permanent teeth to erupt. This could save you future orthodontic bills.
- Beware of baby pacifiers and teething rings that can be easily broken or swallowed. Make sure the shield is not too small or too flexible to prevent the baby's choking or asphyxiation.

ORTHODONTIA

An orthodontist is a dentist who specializes in correcting malocclusion (the improper position of the teeth). There are approximately 6500 orthodontists in the United States. No one knows exactly how many general dentists also do orthodontia*.

How prevalent are orthodontic problems? Several surveys estimate that about 50% of children need some form of orthodontic care, and that 1 in every 5 children suffers a severe malocclusion.

Until recently, many insurance companies excluded orthodontic treatments because they were considered merely "cosmetic." However, the coverage is broadening, and the demand and fees for orthodontia remain high. As insurance plans cover orthodontic treatments more routinely, orthodontia is becoming more available to those who might not have been able to afford it.

Ring Lardner said, "Looks don't mean anything, just ninety percent." We are a nation obsessed with our appearance. Our media constantly spew out ads to look thinner, smell better, and appear sexier. We spend billions of dollars on deodorants, hair dyes, shampoos, shaving creams, nail polish, perfumes, diet products, facial creams, and makeup. Clearly, we *do* care how we look. Plastic surgery, face lifts, nose bobbing, breast contouring, hair transplants, and buttocks restructuring make teeth straightening seem as commonplace as our hairbrush. The face is the most dramatic focus of our appearance, and an attractive smile can light up the face. So it is understandable that anyone who cares about his appearance is concerned about his teeth.

Why are orthodontic fees so high?

Most family dentists do not treat major orthodontic defects because they have not been adequately trained. 50% of children need orthodontic treatments, but there are only 6500 orthodontists. Obviously the demand exceeds the supply. Dental schools traditionally devote only a small amount of time to this subject, and orthodontists often carefully guard who will be admitted and who will be excluded from their courses. Some observers (myself included) believe the orthodontic professors do not wish to reveal too much. This is another

*Orthodontics is the term preferred by many Orthodontists.

case of a "closed shop" that keeps fees high. In effect, they prevent competition from developing. Their policy seems to be quite effective because most general dentists who feel equipped to do some endodontia, periodontia, exodontia, and prosthodontia hesitate to take on orthodontia. Result? Higher fees for you.

If you think your child needs orthodontic attention, ask your family dentist first. If it is a simple movement of a single tooth, he may feel equipped to handle it. If not, he'll refer you to a specialist. If you have heard about an orthodontist by reputation, you may even call him direct.

My child goes to a pedodontist. Can he treat his orthodontic problem, too?

Your pedodontist is in an excellent position to practice *Interceptive orthodontics.* Early detection can prevent severe malocclusions from developing, so your pedodontist can probably pick up and head off a major problem. He can prevent more extensive orthodontic problems by early intervention, using various appliances such as space maintainers, space regainers, and head caps ("night braces"). This could save you money by minimizing or eliminating possible orthodontic bills several years down the line.

Some pedodontists today practice a hybrid dual specialty of orthodontia *and* pedodontia. They fill and maintain your child's teeth as well as construct and insert orthodontic appliances. There is a certain advantage to having both phases of work done by the same dentist, because he takes responsibility for the overall health of your child's mouth. It could cost you less, too.

Musicians and Malocclusion

Does your child play a wind instrument? Cupshaped mouthpieces, such as the trumpet and the trombone, tend to correct "buck teeth," while flute and piccolo tend to increase it. Saxophone players can go either way, and oboe players may find their "buck teeth" reduced and their bite opened.

At what age should my child start orthodontic treatments?

Many specialists believe in waiting until all the permanent teeth (except wisdom teeth) have erupted — around 12 — before starting orthodontia. It simplifies their work because they know exactly how much permanent tooth structure there is compared to the size of the jaw. They contend that certain mechanical techniques are unsuitable when there is a mixed dentition of baby and permanent teeth in the mouth.

Others argue that it is unwise to wait idly while the teeth drift into worse positions. They believe treatments can begin once the six year molars have erupted, and that major therapy can be avoided this way. Simple orthodontic interception techniques* are applied in the hope of averting a full blown problem in the teenage years. Very little can be lost by having your child "evaluated" for orthodontia during his regular checkups. You could save money by investigating *interceptive orthodontia*.

Can orthodontia be started too early?

Yes. Watch out for the orthodontist who puts an appliance in too early, in order to keep you in his practice and prevent you from going elsewhere. This type of orthodontist keeps the patient in a holding pattern until active treatment can begin, perhaps eighteen months later. When that time rolls around, your child's enthusiasm has waned, and he is fed up because there has been no visible improvement. At this point, it's hard to stir up interest and cooperation for active treatment.

If nothing seems to be happening for months after your child's appliance has been inserted, ask why and set up a special consultation. You have that right. Maybe your orthodontist was looking out for himself, not your child.

Why does my child have to have four healthy permanent teeth extracted?

Many orthodontists require four permanent teeth to be removed prior to starting orthodontic banding. This is necessary in cases of

---

*The Denholtz Muscle Anchorage Appliance is one of these. It harnesses lip pressures to move teeth and has been successfully used in children as young as six.

crowding where the child has large teeth and too small a jaw to accommodate them. The teeth are so crowded there simply is not enough room to align them into a proper and pleasing arrangement. Of course, the extraction of four teeth may have an emotional impact on both the parents and the child, who may be reluctant to accept this diagnosis. Before making this diagnosis, the orthodontist should have taken molds of your child's teeth (study models) and cephalometric X rays (a special X ray that indicates the relationship of the bones to the teeth). Not every case requires four extractions, so don't submit meekly. Ask your orthodontist to explain his diagnosis.

Is there any way to avoid four extractions?

There are some orthodontists who remove four teeth in almost every case. Standardization of their techniques makes for a busy, efficient, and lucrative office. But it is certainly more important to consider each patient individually — their unique facial profile and their own personal ideas of beauty. Some people like the toothy Dinah Shore smile. Others prefer a thin lipped, flat, Jacqueline Onassis look. It is not unusual for two orthodontists to disagree on the same case. One insists four teeth must be extracted and the other claims extractions are unnecessary.

A dental consumer cannot play orthodontist but he should be aware of the potential *pitfalls of removing four teeth:*

1. Once teeth are extracted, no reversal of the treatment is possible. You can't put the teeth back in.
2. Sometimes the extraction of four teeth (one in each quadrant) results in *too much* tooth structure removed.
3. Instead of crowding. there is now *too much space* between the teeth, causing "open contacts."
4. Four extractions may produce a "caved in" appearance or an overflattened profile. The nose and chin become too prominent, giving a "little old man or woman" look. (Fig. 8-1).

A highly competent specialist could avoid these pitfalls by pulling the back teeth forward and pushing the front teeth back.

NORMAL PROFILE

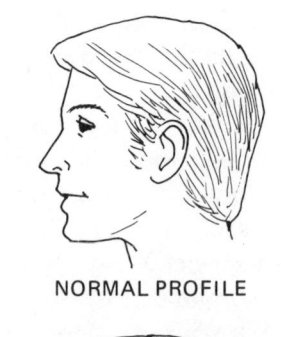

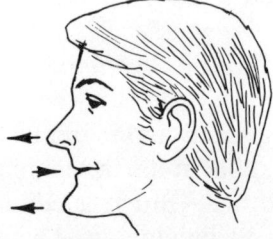

"CAVED IN LOOK"

Four extractions may produce a "CAVED IN APPEARANCE". Nose and chin become too prominent.

Fig. 8-1

Ask your dentist to recommend a *non-extraction oriented orthodontist.* If he, too, concurs that extractions are indeed the only way, then you can be confident about going ahead. *Don't hesitate to get another opinion.* Your dental records are yours if you've paid your bill, so have them forwarded. Duplicating study models are costly, and repeating X rays is unhealthy.

How long do orthodontic treatments take?

On the average, a full blown "four extraction" case could take about two years, give or take six months. The length of treatment depends on the individual case and the cooperation and motivation of the patient. For example, if a patient consistently misses appointments and does not follow instructions, the case will stretch out. If the child forgets to wear his elastics (elastic power generates the force necessary to move teeth), the treatment will stall like a car without gas power. Failure to follow instructions can prolong treatment and contribute to poor results. Cooperative and highly motivated patients could cut the treatment time.

Once the teeth have been straightened, can they become crooked again?

Teeth are set into bone and bone has an "elastic" quality. Therefore, although the teeth have reached the proper position and the braces have been removed, there is a tendency to drift toward the original position. To prevent this, and to "lock" the teeth into place, orthodontic devices called retainers and positioners are used. These can be worn for a year or longer, and the patient can gradually taper off. Unlike braces which are worn all the time, some retainers are worn only at night. It is up to the patient to wear these devices until the teeth are stabilized in their new position.

Do orthodontic treatments hurt?

Generally speaking, orthodontic treatments are painless. Of course everyone's individual pain threshold differs. Most cases are treated by placing metal bands and brackets on the teeth. The initial procedure is usually completed in one or two long visits. There is no drilling, and the procedure consists of fitting the bands and cementing them to the teeth. It may be unpleasant, but it doesn't hurt. Expect to be seen every 2-6 weeks thereafter. Each adjustment visit might require bending a wire, inserting a coil, or adding a spring. The teeth might ache slightly for a day or two. Occasionally, a loose wire may stick into the gum and require attention, but don't let minor irritations deter you if you are genuinely motivated.

How much will it cost?

There is no set fee. Every orthodontic case requires an individual treatment plan, uniquely arrived at for that individual. Most orthodontists prefer to set a fixed fee on a contract basis. A typical $1500 contract might require a $300 deposit and $50 a month for two years. If a retainer is broken or lost, there could be an additional charge of $40-60.

A dental school clinic could charge $800 for a standard two year treatment, for which a private orthodontist charges $1800. A dental school could cut down on your costs, and you will be getting a graduate dentist, not a dental student. Bob G. W. of Oxon Hills, Maryland reports saving money on orthodontic bills. He said, "Having the work done at a university dental school, saved me $1000 on my daughter's teeth." A young orthodontist just starting out might accept $1000 for an $1800 case. Established orthodontists with years of experience are less likely to budge on the fee.

Can malocclusion be harmful to general health?

Yes. If your teeth don't mesh properly like gears, you are probably not chewing your food well. This can put a burden on your digestive system and restrict you to soft foods. Severe malocclusions can affect your jaw muscle, disfigure your facial contours, and perhaps contribute to your jaw "riding" improperly at the temporomandibular joint (in front of the ear), resulting in a constant, dull ache. The emotional impact of impaired speech and appearance can also be psychologically harmful.

Mary Tyler Moore Bucks "Buck Teeth" Image

Mary Tyler Moore, successful TV star, admits how terribly self-conscious she was about her own buck teeth. "Leslie Caron was a big idol of mine," she says. "I identified with her because she had buck teeth, too. I wanted to have my teeth straightened all my life."

What about orthodontia for adults?

Orthodontia is not just for children, and an adult who suffers from a "Bugs Bunny" look can do something about it. A new trend toward adult orthodontia is now becoming acceptable, and even fashionable. Highly visible people — actors, politicians, and teachers — are no longer settling for unattractive mouths. They are seeking orthodontists who will do something about it.

A pet food salesman, Arnold L., tells a typical story. "As a child, my parents couldn't afford to get me braces. My crooked teeth bugged me all my life." Arnold's company recently adopted an insurance plan that will pay $500 toward his orthodontic bill of $1200. His dentist has accepted the $500 as a retainer and Arnold is paying off the balance at $30 a month.

This is no isolated case. A 44 year old New Jersey mother of three is also undergoing orthodontia. Why does she want cosmetic orthodontia at 44? "I plan to go back into the job market now that my kids are grown up. I figure I'll feel more confident with a nice smile."

10% of patients currently undergoing orthodontic treatments are adults. Most of them are women in the 20-40 age bracket. Their motivation is primarily cosmetic, but they are reaping the extra benefits of having functional problems corrected, too. And they're enjoying emotional and psychological dividends along the way.

Are adults self-conscious about wearing braces? A prominent California orthodontist says, "I have had patients in very visible jobs — stewardesses, attorneys in trial work, schoolteachers. Nobody, as far as I know, has had any trouble with employers saying the braces look silly or interfere with their jobs." In the past, adults felt guilty for spending money for "frivolous" or "flimsy" reasons. Today, more and more people are saying "I'm worth it!"

Will I really look a lot better?

Patients who undergo a two year process of orthodontic treatments rarely "see" the change while it is happening, because it is a slow process. But once the bands are off, they are astounded by the dramatic results. When they are shown their "before" models and photographs, their reaction is usually, "Was that me? I can't believe it!"

It's difficult for you to imagine the end result when you decide to begin treatment. Ask your orthodontist to demonstrate on your study models the effect he is working to achieve. Then you'll have a firmer understanding of the benefits.

ORTHODONTIC CONSUMER TIPS

- Don't submit meekly to having four extractions prior to orthodontic treatment.
- Consult a *non-extraction oriented* orthodontist for a second opinion.
- Dont wait until your child is 12 to consider orthodontia.
- Have your child evaluated for *interceptive orthodontia* during his regular checkups.
- A university orthodontic clinic could save you money.
- Adult orthodontia can bring tremendous cosmetic and psychological benefits.
- If you're hesitant about the benefits because you can't visualize the results, ask your orthodontist to show you, *on your study models,* how you will look.

ENDODONTIA

An endodontist is a specialist who limits his practice exclusively to root canal therapy. There are approximately 600 endodontists in the United States, or about 0.5% of all practicing dentists. A great number, perhaps 90% of general dentists, also do root canal therapy. The advantage of using an endodontist is that you are going to an expert who does only this one phase of dentistry. As a result, you can reasonably expect more proficiency and expertise. But the fees will probably be higher. If the root canal appears to be a complicated case, your general dentist will advise you to see an endodontist. In either case, a general rule to follow is: *save the tooth.*

What is root canal therapy?

You have a painful tooth. Your dentist tells you the only way to save it is through root canal therapy. What does that mean? First, your dentist will give you a local anesthetic. He will place a rubber dam (a small rubber mask) around the tooth to isolate it and keep the area dry and uncontaminated. He will make an opening directly into the pulp chamber (completely painless) and remove the diseased nerve and vessels with tiny instruments. (Fig. 8-2) Next, the inside of the root will be cleaned and medicated. These procedures can take one to four visits. After the canal is free from infection and the pain has subsided, it is filled and sealed. Some teeth have only one canal, for example, a front tooth; but a molar could have three or four canals.

When do you need root canal therapy?

A diseased pulp is usually extremely painful. A severe toothache can be a symptom that your tooth requires root canal therapy. Extreme sensitivity to hot and cold can also indicate root canal therapy. Pain on biting may be another clue.
Sometimes deterioration of the nerve is so gradual that no pain symptoms are felt. In that case, a routine X ray exam and other diagnostic techniques can disclose the need for root canal therapy *even when no pain is present.*

156 HOW TO SAVE YOUR TEETH AND YOUR MONEY

Small flexible instrument used to remove, clean, and debride the contents of the root canal.

Decay

Enamel

Pulp chamber

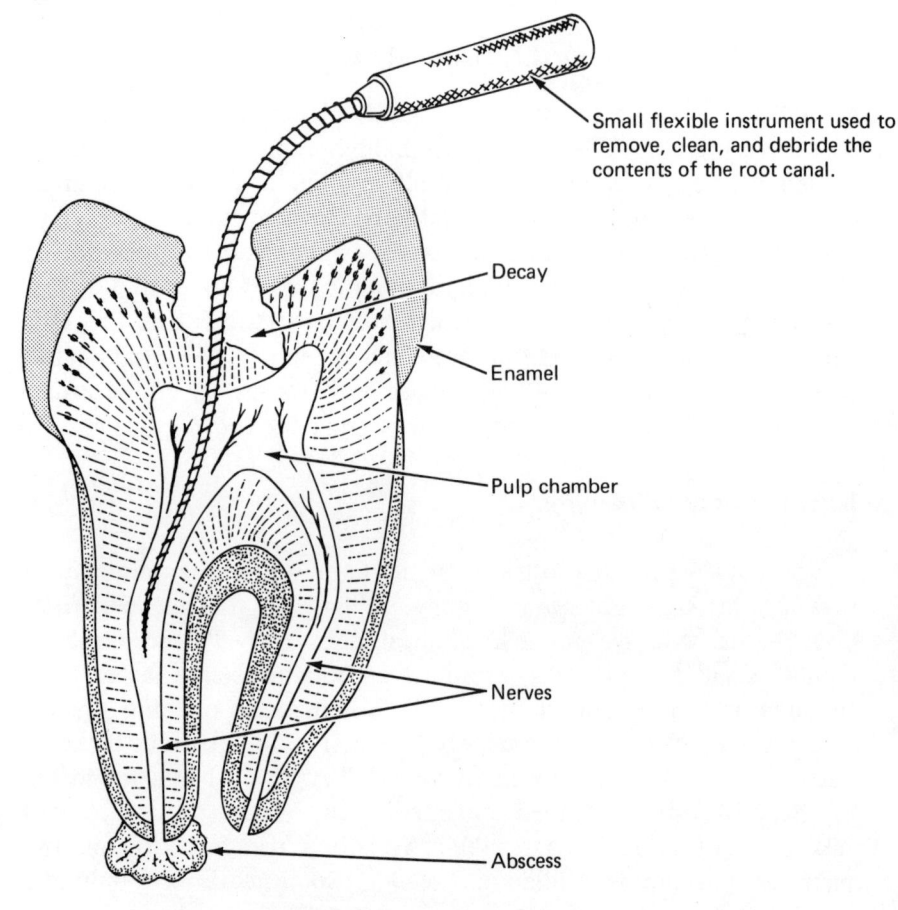

Nerves

Abscess

ROOT CANAL THERAPY
The removal of diseased nerve and vessels with tiny instruments
Fig. 8-2

You might also feel a strange pain, *referred into other teeth* remote from the diseased tooth, or even into the ear. You may think you are experiencing an *earache.* It's possible to believe an upper tooth is the offending one when actually it is the lower tooth. In *all* cases the final diagnosis must be made by your dentist.

What causes a tooth to require root canal therapy?

There are several ways the tooth's nerve can become diseased and require root canal therapy:

1. Bacteria can infect the pulp of a tooth through a *deep cavity* where the decay has reached the nerve.
2. A *sharp blow* to a tooth, as in a car accident or a football game, can damage the nerve and cause it to die.
3. Sometimes *advanced periodontal (gum) disease* may affect the nerve. Then *both* periodontic and endodontic treatments are required.

What are the odds for success?

Research indicates that 90-95% of root canal therapy cases are successful. The odds are heavily stacked in your favor.

Do *not* succumb to the fast and easy way out by having your painful tooth extracted. Make every effort to seek root canal therapy and save your own natural tooth.

Tiger's Toothache Cured by Root Canal Therapy

Kundur, a two year old male Siberian tiger, residing in the Philadelphia Zoo, had root canal therapy for two of his lower canine teeth. Now this member of a rare and endangered species may continue to live a long and healthy life. How does a dentist work on a tiger? VERY CAREFULLY, and AFTER the tiger's been put to sleep with an anesthetic dart.

Is root canal therapy a good investment for a consumer?

A tooth that has had root canal therapy could last you the balance of your life. If it lasts only an additional ten years and the fee was $150, you have "rented" your natural tooth for only $15 a year. This is one of the wisest dental investments you could make. Successful root canal therapy avoids the expense of an extraction and replacement with a false tooth. That could cost you around $600 for a fixed bridge. So the cost of root canal therapy is less than the cost of extracting and replacing your natural tooth with an artificial one.

Is root canal therapy always so simple and painless?

No. Sometimes a tooth does not respond to conventional treatment. In difficult cases (about 10%) it might be necessary to make a small "window" in the gum so that the very tip of the tooth can be reached directly. This is called an *apicoectomy* — removing the tip of the root through the gum. It is more complicated and could cause pain and swelling for a few days. But for those few days of discomfort you could save your tooth for many more years. It's a good investment and may not cost much more than conventional root canal therapy.

Are all my troubles over once the root canal phase has been completed?

No. The canals are completed, but the cavity still has to be filled. Maybe a simple filling is all you're in for. But if the tooth was badly decayed and broken down, a crown may be necessary, adding another $200 to the cost of saving the tooth. Don't let this deter you. Would you have a toe removed if it cost $200 or $300 to save it? Why value a tooth any less? Saving the tooth is still better and cheaper than the cost of extracting and replacing the tooth with a fixed bridge.

Does a tooth turn black after root canal therapy?

Sometimes a tooth can "darken" in color, but it doesn't turn black. A discolored tooth can be lightened by bleaching it from the inside. If this fails, a crown can be made to cover it, thus restoring the original appearance and color.

What are the fees for a root canal?

Fees for root canal therapy are based on the number of canals within the tooth. An average fee for the first canal might be $125. But each additional canal in the same tooth could add another $50 per canal. Therefore, a three rooted back tooth could run $225.*
An endodontist's fees will probably run higher than a general dentist's.

*Some offices may charge as high as $350.

What's a pulp cap?

Sometimes, if the nerve has merely been "touched" by decay, a simple protective sedative can be placed over the nerve exposure. This is called a pulp cap, and it could cost about $25. It *might* eliminate the need for root canal therapy. On the other hand, the tooth could kick up again. But if it works, you've avoided a root canal, additional visits, and a higher dental bill.

● ● ● ● ●

Recently, a controversy in the field of endodontia has come to a head over an alternate method of performing root canal therapy: the Sargenti Technique. Unlike most medical-dental controversies that are discussed exclusively in scientific journals, this one received wide coverage in newspapers and popular magazines like *Newsweek*. What is it all about?

In the conventional method of root canal therapy, the endodontist drills a hole in the crown of the tooth and removes the nerve with various broaches, reamers, and files — a tedious *manual* operation requiring dexterity. After cleaning, the canal is filled with gutta-percha, an inert gumlike material. Treatment may take from one to four visits, and the cost of a single tooth can range from $125 to $350.

The Sargenti Technique, named for the Swiss dentist who introduced it, differs from this conventional method in two ways. First, the dentist uses a small *motorized* device instead of the standard hand instruments, which simplifies the procedure. Secondly, the Sargenti practitioners fill the canal with "N-2," a special paste containing lead, mercury, paraformaldehyde, and steroid hormones. These powerful ingredients, they say, sterilize and protect the root canal from further bacterial growth. The N-2 formula has changed several times.

What does all this mean to you, the dental consumer? The Sargenti Technique can be completed in one or two visits, and costs as little as $50. So it cuts down time and money. Can *any* dentist do it? After a one day course, the general dentist can learn this technique and become a member of The American Endodontic Society.*

---

*Dr. John I. Ingle of Washington says, "The AES claims that 20,000 U.S. dentists have taken the N2 courses. At $100 tuition, that comes to $2,000,000, which has evidently been split among the three or four leaders of the AES who serve as the primary instructors. If it isn't split this way, where is the money going?"

On the other hand, conventional endodontists (members of The American Association of Endodontists) and some general dentists contend the Sargenti Technique is *not effective and could be dangerous.* They claim the motorized technique is not thorough in removing all remnants of nerve and pulp tissue, and the filling material N-2 is hazardous. They say the paste N-2, containing lead and mercury compounds, poses a toxic hazard, and that the formaldehyde (commonly used as embalming fluid) is damaging to the tissue. California, Australia, Norway, and Sweden have banned the drug, and some Sargenti practitioners have been the target of malpractice suits. One recent malpractice suit contended that the patient had to be hospitalized and receive plastic surgery because the roof of her mouth had sloughed away following treatment.

Sargenti proponents say their paste is safe and cuts down time, pain, and costs for the patient. But the United States Food and Drug Administration has not approved it, and an outright ban may be in the making. The controversy has even reached the halls of Congress. One representative reported that "the poisons, including lead and embalming fluid, can reach the vital organs and bone marrow."

In any case, opt for root canal therapy and save your tooth.

ENDODONTIC CONSUMER TIPS

- A painful tooth does *not* necessarily require an extraction.
- It's good consumerism to try to save the tooth with root canal therapy.
- The cost of root canal therapy depends on the number of canals, so a front tooth is less expensive than a back tooth.
- Root canal therapy could cost from $50 (Sargenti) to $350 (conventional), but extracting a tooth and replacing it with a fixed bridge could cost $600.
- A badly decayed tooth may require a crown to support it *after* root canal therapy. Ask your dentist if you'll need one.
- If a tooth "darkens" after root canal therapy, ask about "bleaching" it.
- If the nerve has only been "touched," ask your dentist about a pulp cap ($25) instead of root canal therapy.
- The Sargenti Technique is faster and cheaper, but there are *risks* involved.
- Ask your dentist if he uses the Sargenti Technique or traditional root canal therapy, before you decide what to do.

PERIODONTIA

A periodontist is a dentist who limits his practice to the treatment of the gums, bones, and supporting tissue that hold the teeth in place. Although many general dentists will treat less complicated gum disorders, a periodontist is the one to see when gum surgery is necessary.* If you think that having cavity free teeth means no dental bills, you're mistaken. Gum disease is nearly a universal ailment. It strikes 95% of the population at one time or another, and *after 35 it is the chief cause of loss of teeth.*

What is periodontal disease?

Periodontal disease involves problems of the gums, bones, and supporting tissue that surround the teeth. Most people are unaware that they have gum problems, because the disease develops slowly and insidiously, and unlike a toothache is not usually painful. As people get older gum problems set in; so now that we are living longer, the incidence of periodontal disease is increasing. Many people tend to accept this passively as just another symptom of aging. They think gum problems go along with greying hair and wrinkles, and there's not much they can do about it. They are wrong!

How can you tell if you have periodontal disease?

Symptons of periodontal disease tend to be overlooked. Here are the warning signs. You should check with your dentist if you have them:

1. Puffy, flabby, red, or swollen gums.
2. Bleeding gums when you brush your teeth, use dental floss, or eat.
3. Persistent bad breath (halitosis).
4. Loosening of your teeth.
5. Spaces developing between your teeth, allowing your teeth to "migrate" or shift.

*There were 1,114 periodontists in 1973, excluding the Armed Forces.

What is the primary cause of periodontal disease?

The primary cause of gum troubles is plaque. Dental plaque is a sticky, transparent film of bacteria, saliva, and debris that accumulates on the teeth. If the plaque is not removed by daily toothbrushing and flossing, it can harden into a crusty deposit called calculus (tartar). The calculus acts as an irritant, then wedges the gums away from the roots of the teeth forming *pockets* (spaces between the roots of the teeth and the gums). (Fig. 8-3). As these pockets become deeper, they fill with more bacteria, food debris, and pus. This causes the gums to become red, puffy, sore, and to bleed. If left untreated, these pockets become deeper, and the bone that

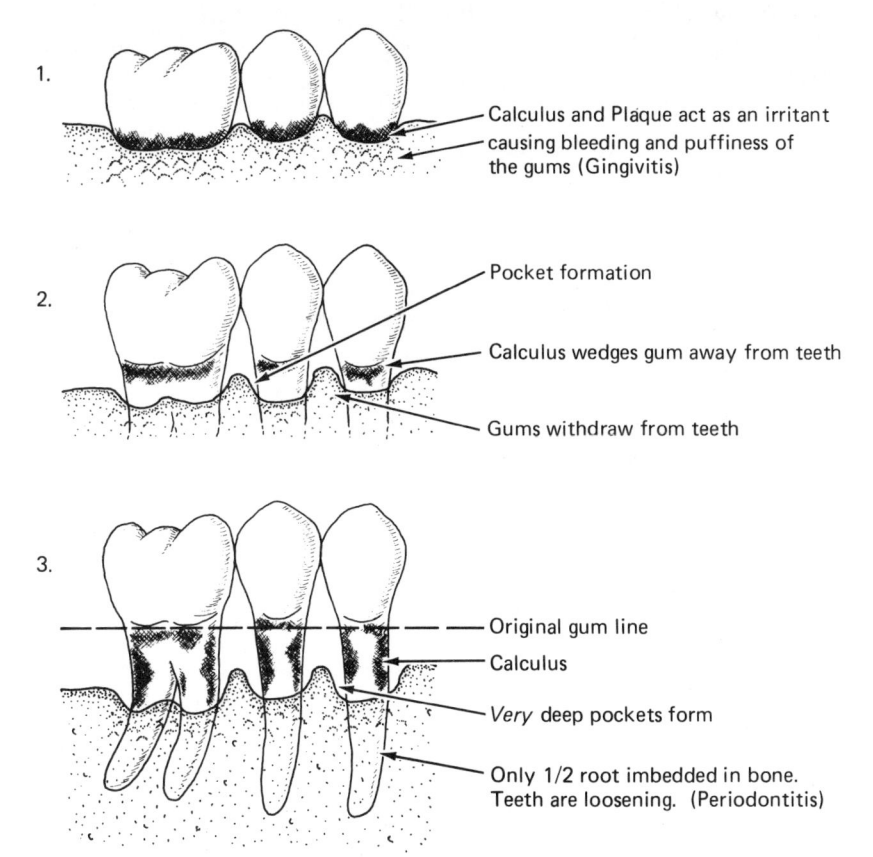

1. Calculus and Plaque act as an irritant causing bleeding and puffiness of the gums (Gingivitis)

2. Pocket formation
   Calculus wedges gum away from teeth
   Gums withdraw from teeth

3. Original gum line
   Calculus
   Very deep pockets form
   Only 1/2 root imbedded in bone. Teeth are loosening. (Periodontitis)

Fig. 8-3

supports the teeth is also attacked. Consequently, the teeth become looser and looser and, in the end, they may have to come out.

Just as a house built on a poor foundation can crumble, healthy teeth can be lost if the supporting structure disintegrates. You *can* lose healthy teeth through periodontal disease. Freedom from cavities does *not* guarantee good dental health.

How can I eliminate dental plaque?

Since plaque is colorless and transparent, it's hard to see. It helps to "disclose" or color the plaque to determine exactly where it is located on the teeth. Ask your dentist about disclosing tablets (or solutions). They're easy to use at home, inexpensive, and they'll help you check to see if you've missed any spots while brushing or flossing. Here is how they work:

1. *After* you've brushed and flossed your teeth, chew a tablet.
2. Spit or swallow (the disclosing dye is harmless) to empty your mouth.
3. Examine your teeth in the mirror under a good light.* The stained area you see is plaque.
4. Rebrush and then use dental floss to get in between the teeth until all the stains are removed.
5. Do this daily. After a while, you can cut down on the disclosing tablets to once a week.

If you are plaque free on a daily basis, you are on the road to healthier gums and teeth. This means lower dental bills for you.

Are there other factors in addition to plaque that cause gum disease?

Yes. Other local irritants in the mouth can also contribute to gum disease. An imperfectly contoured filling or crown can be a factor, as can a poor fitting partial denture. Malocclusion, mouth breathing, and bruxism (grinding the teeth together during sleep) can also contribute. So can the destructive habits of using bobby pins or

---

*There are special plaque lights, with mirrors, that you can keep in your bathroom.

toothpicks, which can irritate your gums. The hormonal changes during pregnancy and menopause may also produce puffy, swollen gums.

> **Bleeding Gums and the Pill**
>
> *Bleeding gums can result from unusual reasons. In* "The Doctor's Case Against The Pill," *Barbara Seaman states that some of the women interviewed reported post-Pill complaints. Hair loss and bleeding gums were among their problems when they stopped using the Pill.*

Are there different kinds of gum disease?

Yes. Periodontal problems develop in two stages. The early stage is called *gingivitis* and is an inflammation of the gums. This is characterized by mild redness along the margins of the gum and a tendency toward bleeding. The later stage, *periodontitis ("pyorrhea")*, is the advanced stage in which the gums and underlying bone are also attacked. Your own family dentist might pick up your early stage of gingivitis. At this point you can do something to prevent advanced periodontitis, which could cause you to lose all your teeth. The majority of people in this country allow perfectly healthy teeth to be extracted, and wind up wearing dentures when their teeth might have been saved. Periodontitis can cause you to lose perfectly healthy teeth.

What is the treatment for gum disease?

Gum disease can be treated. Mild cases of gingivitis may respond to a simple prophylaxis or deep scaling. The objective is to remove the plaque and calculus which cause the local gum irritation. This could be followed by a minor surgical treatment called *curettage.* *
If this conservative approach is successful (coupled with scrupulous home care) you could avoid complicated and expensive surgery.

*Scraping of soft tissue of the gum.

On the other hand, advanced periodontitis cases will require surgical techniques, such as recontouring and "tightening" the gums or grafting tissue from one part of the mouth to another. *Gingivectomy,* the removal of gum tissue, and *gingivoplasty,* reshaping the gums, may be necessary.

If the bone supporting the teeth has also been attacked, then bone surgery will be called for. The periodontist may perform an *osteoplasty,* which means reshaping the bone around the teeth. This is even more complicated than gum surgery. It requires "flapping," or peeling back the gum tissue, recontouring the bone, then sewing the gum tissue back. *Bone transplants* could also be used in which a small "plug" of bone is transplanted from one site to another.

How much will it cost and how long will it take?

Like orthodontic treatments, periodontic treatments are designed according to each individual's needs. Therefore, the length of time and the costs depend on the extent of the disease. If conservative procedures like scaling and curettage are used, the costs ($20-40 per visit) will be less than a full blown surgical treatment which could run $1000-2000 or more, depending on the extent of the surgery. A curettage is obviously less expensive than an involved osteoplasty or bone transplant, which could require months of treatment.

In a typical surgical case, the periodontist might treat one quadrant of the mouth at a time with visits of perhaps an hour each. He might perform the surgery, then ask you to return in one week to change the dressing. Surgical packs, wires, or splints may be used to stabilize the teeth between visits. The front teeth may be done in separate additional visits. Treatment involving *all* the teeth could take six months or longer.

In both simple and surgical cases, the periodontist should also design an individual plan for your home care, which could include disclosing tablets for plaque control, dental floss, and an interdental stimulator for the gums. He may advise you to wear a bite plate if you grind your teeth at night, and he may also equilibrate your bite.

In all cases, simple or complicated, you must return for regular checkups over a period of months, to evaluate your progress and to reinforce your home care.

Is it painful to have periodontal treatments?

With the use of local anesthetics, you should not experience pain during the surgery. However, you may experience post-operative pain and swelling for 1-3 days after the surgery. Your dentist will probably prescribe pills to relieve the pain and make you comfortable.

What is "trench mouth?"

"Trench mouth" is a layman's term for an acute and painful infection that mainly attacks the gums, but can spread to parts of the mouth and throat. It was dubbed "trench mouth" during World War I when many soldiers suffered from it. Although it frequently occurs in a group of people living under the same conditions, it has not been shown to be contagious, as many people believe. It is also known as Vincent's Infection, or more correctly as Necrotizing Ulcerative Gingivitis (NUG). The symptoms include a foul odor, ulceration and bleeding of the gums, extreme pain, excessive salivation, and even an elevation in body temperature. Contributing factors are poor diet, smoking, physical or mental stress, and very poor oral hygiene.

A *canker sore* is a small ulcer in the lining of the mouth, and should not be mistaken for "trench mouth." It is probably caused by a virus. A *cold sore* on the lip will heal in 8-10 days, with or without treatment. When a patient asks, "What can I do about this sore on my lip?" the dentist might reply, "It will take about 7 days to heal if you leave it alone. If I treat it, it will only last a week."

PERIODONTAL CONSUMER TIPS

- The largest single cause of periodontal disease is plaque, which eventually can destroy the gums and bones that support your teeth.
- Ask your dentist if you have periodontal problems *at each checkup*. Healthy teeth can loosen up and be lost if periodontal disease sets in. *You could lose all your teeth.*
- For periodontal treatments to be effective, it is absolutely necessary to institute a thorough oral hygiene routine at home.
- Become a *co-therapist* with your dentist by using disclosing tablets and removing plaque on a daily basis. It's inexpensive and can cut your dental bills.
- Have a professional prophylaxis by your dentist or oral hygienist on a regular 3-6 month basis. This is a sound dental investment and should not be skipped.
- Do not allow a mild *gingivitis* to turn into an advanced *periodontitis* that requires expensive and complicated surgery.
- It is useless to have expensive periodontal treatments unless you are highly motivated to *protect your investment* at home.
- Don't waste your money on "cold sore" cures.

PROSTHODONTIA

A prosthodontist is a dentist who limits his practice to replacing missing teeth with artificial (prosthetic) teeth. Practically every general dentist also does prosthetic work for his patients, and therefore, there are only a small number of prosthodontists.* These specialists are usually referred the "impossible" cases that the general dentist does not wish to be involved with. An example would be an edentulous patient who requires a denture, but has a flat or totally "resorbed" ridge. This type of problem is so difficult that the patient may have already discarded five or six unsuccessful dentures. He might even show a bagful to his general dentist, who concludes the best choice for this patient would be to see the prosthodontist.

If you need to have teeth replaced, your dentist will probably explain to you that there are two types of artificial replacements, *removable* and *fixed*. Removable means the patient can easily take the artificial teeth in and out of his mouth. Fixed means the artificial teeth are permanently cemented into place and cannot be removed by the patient. Removable replacements conjure up the unpleasant picture of "false teeth" soaking in a glass of water on the bedside nightstand. Is that accurate? What's the difference between fixed and removable replacements? Which is better? Which costs more (or less)? Which feels better? Looks better? Lasts longer? What are the advantages and disadvantages of each?

First of all, if you have *no teeth* in the upper jaw or lower jaw, *you have no choice.*** There's nothing to cement false teeth *to,* so you can only have removable work. This is called a *full denture.* If you have no upper teeth, you will need a *full upper denture;* if you have no lower teeth, you will need a *full lower denture.* Your own dentist can probably do this for you, unless there is a special problem.

Don't select stark white teeth. Natural teeth are somewhat yellow, irregular, and even stained as we get older. If you want your denture to look natural, the artificial teeth should have slight imperfections and rotations. A row of gleaming white chicklets in perfect alignment is a dead giveaway.

---

*There were 702 prosthodontists in 1973, excluding the Armed Forces.
**With the exception of implants, pp. 189 and 213.

> **Teeth Like Pearls? Never**
>
> *When people in Thailand lose a tooth, do they select a pearly white false tooth? No. They prefer a black tooth to match their natural teeth, which are often stained black from betel nuts. To replace a lost tooth with a white tooth would look strange.*

But suppose you still have *some* teeth in your mouth — a few in the lower jaw and a few in the upper jaw — *then you have a choice.* You can choose:

1. A *removable* appliance called "a partial denture."
2. A *fixed* appliance called "a fixed bridge."

The Partial Denture

A partial denture is a removable appliance that replaces missing teeth, when you still have some natural teeth in your mouth. It is usually held in place by clasps (hooks) that encircle several of your remaining natural teeth. The partial can be snapped in and out easily. The removable partial denture is the *most common* method of replacing missing teeth. Why? Because it costs considerably *less money* than fixed bridgework. Here's how it works.

If you select a removable denture, the cost will not vary much whether you require two teeth or eight teeth replaced. But in a fixed bridge, you will be charged for *each tooth replacement by the unit.* A removable denture replacing eight teeth could cost you only $250. But to replace the same eight teeth with fixed bridgework could run $2400, about ten times as much. Why? Your dentist might charge $200 *per unit,* times eight missing teeth (units), equals $1600. Add to that four additional units to anchor the false teeth to the natural teeth (4 × $200 = $800), and you're up to $2400.

Why is there such a huge disparity between the fee for fixed and removable replacements? In a removable replacement, the dentist takes impressions in one visit. The removable is made of stainless steel and plastic, and the dentist's lab fee is relatively low. But the fixed bridge takes multiple, longer visits *to cut down and prepare each tooth individually.* It requires greater skill, and a *special impression must be made for each tooth.* In addition to the extra time and individual work and skill, fixed bridges are made of precious metal and the lab fees to the dentist are many times higher. Assuming you can afford to spend $2400, is it worth it? Is fixed bridgework better fitting, longer lasting, better looking? Let's look at some of the facts.

In spite of the cheaper costs to the patient (maybe one tenth the fee of fixed bridgework) there is a trend *away from* the cheaper removable partial denture. Why? First, as dental insurance plans are increasing, more dental consumers can afford fixed bridgework. Next, dental consumers are becoming more informed and demanding better quality appliances. Lastly, there is a recognition of the superiority of fixed bridgework. **What are the disadvantages of the removable partial denture?**

1. The psychological and emotional impact of taking your teeth in and out is a constant reminder that your teeth are indeed "false." You can lose them or drop them each time you take them out.
2. Food tends to collect and lodge around the clasps, causing odors. Some patients report the feeling of "denture mouth."
3. The clasps or hooks could hasten decay in the natural end teeth that serve as an anchor for the artificial teeth, unless scrupulous oral hygiene is practiced at home. If you wear removable partial dentures, it is essential that you see your dentist regularly to preserve these valuable remaining teeth.
4. Partial removable dentures are bulky and can be a nuisance. In some cases patients complain that they contribute to garbled speech. Some patients simply can *not* adapt to a "foreign body" in their mouth and wear their dentures in their bureau drawer.
5. The metal clasps* can "loosen up" and cause the partial to ride up or down while eating. They can irritate gums.
6. Even the best made partials have a certain amount of "normal" shift and movement during chewing, and this can be clumsy and limit your selection of foods.

---

*"Precision attachments," a more expensive version of a partial denture, eliminate the clasps. Instead, a male prong fits into a female groove built into the crowned tooth, resulting in an improved appearance and efficiency.

The Full Denture

If you think partial removable dentures can be a problem, what about full dentures — "uppers" or "lowers" when you have *no* natural teeth left? Full dentures are the second kind of *removable* prosthetic appliances. Sometimes called "plates," they are *the last resort when all your teeth have been removed.* Don't buy that phony story that all your dental problems will be over once you wear dentures. On the contrary, for many people, these artificial appliances are the ultimate failure, representing loss of youth, loss of sexual powers, and loss of vitality.

> **Toothless at 65**
>
> *More than half of the people in the United States have lost all their teeth by the time they reach 65. By the time these Senior Citizens reach 75, nearly two-thirds are totally without teeth. It looks like the* golden age *is also the* toothless age *for many Americans.*

Maybe you've heard the horror stories of the full denture. Are they true? **What causes a patient's dissatisfaction with "plates?"**

1. The uppers tend to drop down and the lowers tend to ride up, making clicking *noises* and causing terribly *embarrassing moments.*
2. Full dentures can *feel large and bulky* in your mouth, an uncomfortable foreign body that's unnatural and clumsy. It's hard to get used to them and, *at best,* they cannot approach the natural feeling of your own teeth.
3. It's harder to chew with full dentures, and you are *severely limited in what you can eat.* In spite of the flamboyant claims of denture adhesives on television ads, full denture wearers tend to shy away from biting into an apple. This simple pleasure is lost, and the best they can do is cut the apple into small pieces to make it manageable. Psychologically, that's demoralizing. An adult is reduced to a child whose *food must be cut into bite size pieces.*

4. Denture wearers learn to "like" soft manageable foods like mashed potatoes, hash, and stew. They avoid nuts, crusty rye breads, and corn on the cob, and they *seek out a diet that is easier to chew.* They choose a hamburger over steak simply because they can't manage a steak.
5. Full denture wearers lose a lot of their sense of taste. The plastic of an "upper," for example, covers the roof of the mouth so the taste buds located there are covered, too. This causes foods to taste alike. Spicy foods and bland foods, and hot foods and cold foods are blunted into a dreadful sameness. Since sensitivity is diminished and taste blunted, the *real joy of eating is greatly diminished.*
6. Since there are no natural teeth to anchor the full dentures into place, they tend to rock and shift or even drop while eating. Denture *sore spots* can develop from this sliding and slipping, and *eating efficiency can be lowered* as much as 80%.

    It has been estimated that people with natural teeth can register 125 pounds of biting force, but those wearing dentures register 25-45 pounds. That's a tremendous loss in eating efficiency.
7. Dentures need periodic upkeep and repair to adjust for changes in mouth tissue and jawbones, and for the general wear and tear on the false teeth. Don't expect them to last forever.
8. Dentures should be cleaned after every meal with a denture brush and denture paste or toothpaste. If you want to cut costs, baking soda and regular soap will work as well. But in addition, you should soak your dentures for 15 minutes every week.
9. Overuse of adhesive powders to keep poorly fitting plates from shifting can irritate gums and soft tissues of the mouth. causing tenderness and pain.
10. Dentures settle over the years and facial tissues sag. If you are a denture wearer considering plastic surgery for cosmetic improvement, see your dentist first. He may wish to build up your dentures and restore facial contours.

What are *immediate dentures?* Shouldn't you wait six months after the extractions heal before having plates fitted? Immediate dentures are full uppers and lowers that are inserted into the patient's mouth the *same day the teeth are extracted.* There is no additional discomfort. As a matter of fact, more and more dentists are suggesting that waiting six months is *not* advisable. Some wait a few weeks, but there are definite advantages to immediate dentures. Obviously, you won't have to walk around toothless. If you are employed, that can be important to you. You can go right back to work without suffering the indignity of appearing on the job without teeth, with your face collapsed and your ego deflated. Immediate dentures eliminate the embarrassing waiting period.

However, immediate dentures tend to "loosen up." The gum and bone usually shrink after the extractions, but the denture doesn't change its shape, so the plate may not fit as well in two or three months. At that time you can have it "relined." That means reusing the same false teeth, but putting additional plastic inside the plate to take up the slack. Otherwise, you will need a complete new denture. *A reline should be adequate and cost a lot less than a second set of plates.* You could spend $50-75 for a reline, but a new upper or lower plate could run $250 or more.

Watch out for the tantalizing offers of "extraction mills." They make immediate dentures for $40-50, but you can inherit a whole bagful of troubles along with them. Kenneth Cohen, a dental student at Emory University School of Dentistry, reports that his dental clinic is getting patients who come to have those cheap dentures *remade because they are unusable.* After paying about $50, one woman brought in her cheap dentures because she couldn't wear them. Cohen says, "In Florence, South Carolina, there's a big outfit* that has a lot of lab technicians and employs a couple of dentists. It's a one day deal — you're in the parking lot at 5 A.M. and out that afternoon with a set of dentures. It's a huge operation. Apparently, what they do is snap off a couple of quick impressions and go from there. They're putting in a lot of plates."

One woman brought her cheap dentures into the dental school clinic and Cohen says, "they looked perfectly fine when I held them in my hand. But when she tried to use them, they didn't work and didn't fit." This clinic sees a lot of those people who were duped by cheap dentures. "The impetus is to save money."

*The Sexton Shealey Clinic.

If you, too, are trying to save money, avoid the extraction mills. Avoid the dentist who "sells" plates as a panacea and gladly extracts any teeth in your mouth. It can happen to you, too.

A midwestern dentist extracted nine remaining teeth from a 32 year old woman to make her an upper denture. A review by insurance examiners showed she had only needed fillings and a partial bridge. "The nine extracted teeth were perfectly sound. This was a mutilation."

Watch out for unnecessary extractions to "sell" plates and bridges. The Pennsylvania Insurance Department reports, "probably 6,000,000 teeth are removed each year that should have been saved." Why? Dr. Max Schoen of the Stony Brook School of Dental Medicine says, "After all, it's cheaper, simpler, and involves less painful work than saving them." Another dentist says, "It takes a moment to pull a tooth, but a filling could take more than 30 times longer. If the fee is basically the same for both jobs, you can see why some dentists are extraction oriented." Besides, replacing teeth after you've pulled them is more lucrative for the dentist than filling teeth.

All things considered, if you *have to* have full dentures, *don't* look for a bargain and *do* expect a period of adjustment. False teeth can *never* approach the functional quality of your own natural teeth. But you *can* learn to live with them, to chew cautiously, and to accept the disadvantages patiently while you're striving to adjust. If your attitude is realistic, you can wear full dentures effectively for many, many years.

Geiger Counter on Call

Tests by the Food and Drug Administration reveal that some dentures may be radioactive. How did that come about? The FDA believes that uranium, used in false teeth to simulate the fluorescent quality of natural teeth, could emit more radiation than the recommended level. How widespread is this? Perhaps 50 million Americans may be wearing these radioactive teeth — the cost of a lustrous smile.

The important consumer lessons to be learned are to *avoid* extractions of your own natural teeth, to *save* your own natural teeth, and *never never* to allow a dentist to extract your teeth to "sell" you a cheap denture. Extraction mills which "sell" you a denture for $40-50, also "sell" extractions. *Don't ever have a healthy tooth taken out.* *

Even root tips and badly broken teeth can sometimes provide enough anchorage for an "overdenture." This is essentially a full denture, but one that clips or plugs on right over those broken natural teeth which have been covered by gold. An "overdenture" can give you a more natural feel than a conventional denture. Why? Because your own natural root tips transfer tactile sensations directly into your bone. That makes the "overdenture" feel more "real."

A Fixed Bridge

Unlike partial or full dentures which can come in and out of your mouth (removable), a fixed bridge is permanently cemented to the remaining teeth in your mouth. If you don't have enough remaining teeth properly positioned, you might not be able to have a fixed bridge, because the artificial teeth have to be "anchored" to your own teeth. Ideally, a fixed bridge is used to replace only a few missing teeth. The artificial teeth are fabricated and then attached to your own natural teeth by means of abutment crowns. This means your natural teeth act as anchors for the false ones. How? The natural teeth are ground down to stubs and crowned to support the fixed bridgework. Remember, your dentist figures these as "units," and charges according to the number of units, so replacing two missing teeth would be a minimum of four units.

There are many advantages to a fixed bridge, but *it is much more expensive.* You should know that it takes a lot more grinding (not painful) and chairtime, too. But in the end, you will have a considerably superior result.

You may wonder: why bother spending a lot of money to replace a missing tooth or teeth? Why not save the money and forget about it? That's *not* a wise decision. It could cost you a lot of progressive dental decay, periodontal disease, malocclusion, temporomandibular joint pain, and cosmetic facial defects. It could also cost you *a lot more money.*

What are the consequences of *not* replacing a missing tooth? (Fig. 8-4)

*With certain exceptions, p. 190.

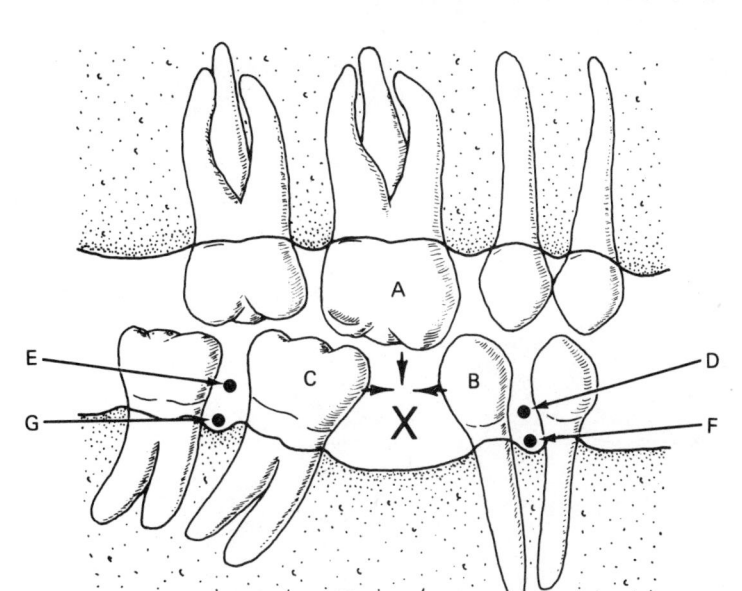

Consequences of **NOT** replacing a missing tooth.
Fig. 8-4

1. The tooth (A) directly above the missing tooth (X) elongates into the space.
2. Adjacent teeth (B and C) drift toward each other into the space.
3. Spaces D and E develop between *B and its adjacent tooth* and *C and its adjacent tooth,* causing "open contacts" for food impaction areas.
4. This, in turn, can contribute to periodontal pockets and bone problems at points F and G.
5. The drifting of teeth can cause malocclusion or improper bite, which decreases chewing efficiency.
6. Faulty bite can contribute to strain on the jaw joint and muscles and produce possible temporomandibular joint pain, experienced as a "headache" in front of the ears.
7. A single missing tooth contributes to the drifting of additional teeth inducing periodontal problems in other areas.
8. Missing teeth can produce a "caved in face" or other cosmetic defects.

178 HOW TO SAVE YOUR TEETH AND YOUR MONEY

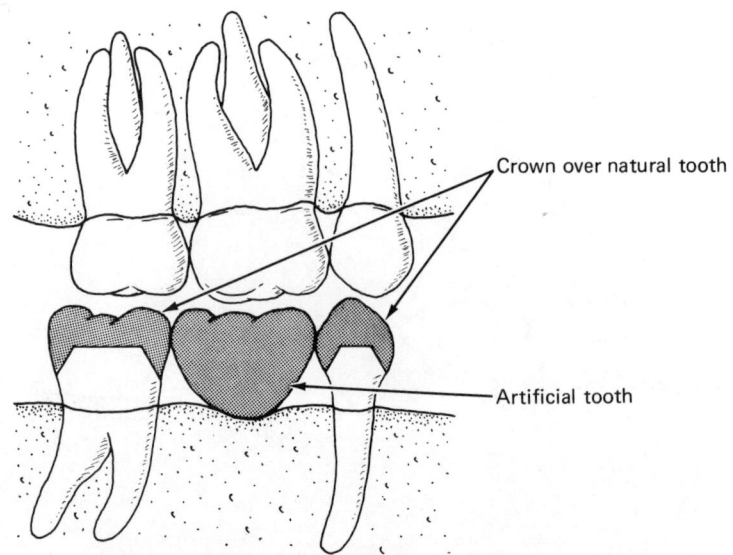

Crown over natural tooth

Artificial tooth

Replacement of One Missing Tooth with a 3 Unit Fixed Bridge.

Fig. 8-5

A properly constructed fixed bridge replacing a single missing tooth (Fig. 8-5) could cost about $600 ($200 a unit × 3). It could also eliminate high costs of periodontal treatments and additional replacements later on.

What are the advantages of a fixed bridge over a partial removable denture?

It costs a lot more, so will you be getting a sufficiently superior replacement to warrant spending all that money? A fixed bridge *is* a good buy for the money. Here's why.

1. Since it cannot be removed, you cannot lose it or break it like a partial denture.
2. It's not bulky. It feels so natural in your mouth that after a few weeks, you'll forget which ones are the false teeth and which are your own.
3. It requires no special denture pastes, adhesives, powders, or soaps. You treat fixed bridgework just like your own teeth and brush them as your own.

4. It doesn't interfere with speech or eating. It is a strong permanent replacement and feels good.
5. You can taste your foods exactly as before. The pleasure of eating is not diminished one iota.
6. You can eat anything – chew a steak or bite into corn on the cob. There's no embarrassment about teeth that drop or click.
7. A fixed bridge makes teeth less susceptible to decay than a partial denture and rarely causes gum irritations or any discomfort, because it can't slide around in your mouth.
8. A fixed bridge lasts longer, is more comfortable and trouble free, and requires almost no adjustment period on your part.
9. A fixed bridge is more attractive. Your appearance will not be marred by clasps (as in partials), and you'll probably even look better than before.

Are there any disadvantages? Yes. Obviously the greatest disadvantage is the initial cost. A fixed bridge is expensive. Then, too, if you need an additional false tooth, it can't be added on as in a partial There's a lot of grinding and chair time necessary for the preparation, so elderly or handicapped people might prefer the partial which is faster and cheaper at the outset. But all things considered, if you can afford a fixed bridge, it is certainly far superior to the removable kind.

Crowns, Caps, and Jackets

Maybe you've heard someone comment about a Hollywood movie star, "That smile cost him $5000. He's got a mouthful of jacket crowns." Then you already know that crowning teeth is expensive. A crown – also called a *cap* or a *jacket* – is essentially the same idea as a "unit" of fixed bridgework.

Hollywood Smiles

Realistic portrayals in the movies are often due to the contribution of the dentist. Dr. Henry R. Dwork reports on the "plumpers" made for Marlon Brando in "The Godfather." Other illusions are to age a person or to create special effects, as in "The Exorcist." Jane Alexander, who played Eleanor Roosevelt in the "Eleanor and Franklin" TV Special, received a final touch to her brilliant portrayal with "a little veneer of six front teeth, bigger than my own, which simply snapped into place."

When is a crown necessary?

If you have a tooth that is so badly decayed, with extensive damage on several surfaces, your dentist might suggest a crown to support it functionally. That's one reason to get a crown. Another is to improve your appearance — a simple cosmetic decision because you want to look better. A third reason for a crown could be to act as a support or "anchor" for a fixed bridge.

In each one of these three cases, the natural tooth must be prepared to receive the crown that will be fitted over it. That means the dentist will grind down your natural tooth to a stub, then fit the artificial crown or "cap" over it, covering your own natural tooth stub underneath.

Does the grinding for crowns hurt?

There is no pain since you will be anesthetized. However, the long appointments can be tiring. Here are three tips for your comfort while you are going through extensive crown or fixed bridgework.

1. Crowns require sitting in the dental chair for long periods of time with your mouth stretched wide open. Ask your dentist or the assistant to smear Nivea Creme or Vaseline over your lips to prevent cracking.
2. If you find it tiring to hold your mouth wide open for long periods of time, ask for a rest period now and then, so you can close your mouth. A brief 30-second pause with your mouth closed can relieve that tired jaw and make you more comfortable. Don't suffer in silence because you don't want to waste your dentist's time. You're entitled to be made comfortable.
3. Another small but useful aid to your comfort when you are having extensive grinding is earplugs — either plain earplugs or the ones that pipe in music. Some dentists themselves wear earplugs to prevent a hearing loss from the constant daily highpitched wizz of their drills.

Are there different kinds of crowns?

Crowns can be made of many materials. Gold is recommended for the back (posterior) teeth because gold is stronger. Crowns for front (anterior) teeth are usually a combination of gold plus a facade or "veneer" made of plastic or porcelain over it for appearance sake. The porcelain is generally more desirable because of its superior light reflection and refraction. Also, plastic crowns tend to lose detail and color over the years. Porcelain "jacket crowns" are the most intricate to fabricate, and therefore cost more.

What do crowns cost?

All-gold crowns are usually the least expensive. Gold with an acrylic (plastic) veneer is more expensive. And gold with an all porcelain covering is the most expensive and, of course, the most aesthetic. In cases where cosmetic appearance is of primary concern (as in the case of a television singer who is constantly subjected to close-ups by the camera), all porcelain crowns are made without any gold, to eliminate any possible opaqueness.

A Very Expensive False Tooth

Diamonds may be a girl's best friend, but singer Mick Jagger likes them, too. Reportedly, he has had a diamond set into his front tooth. How's that for insuring a sparkling smile?

Crowns can range from $125 to about $300. They are superb restorations, but watch out for the dentist who *always* pushes crowns over fillings. Ask him if a filling will do as well. Perhaps your dentist can add "retentive pins" which reinforce the filling. A silver filling on three surfaces, with retentive pins, might cost as much as $40. But a crown could run $200, so if you can get an equally good filling, you may not need a crown. On the whole a crown will last longer, so it's a better investment if you can afford it.

Also watch out for the shady dentist who pushes crowns and neglects the rest of your mouth. One dentist charged a woman $4447 for extensive crown and bridgework. Eight months later, abscesses developed and most of her teeth loosened, because he failed to treat her gum disease first.

If you have a decayed tooth that is not extensive enough to warrant a crown, what types of fillings are available?

There are three common types of permanent fillings:

1. a silver filling
2. a white filling
3. a gold filling (inlay)

The *silver filling* (amalgam) is the most common filling material. It is used primarily for routine fillings of back teeth. The drawbacks to it are: it does not have a good edge strength; it is somewhat brittle; and it can crack. If you've just had a silver filling put in, do *not* eat for several hours until it sets. You may find it sensitive to hot and cold for several days.

The *white filling* is used primarily for front teeth because it looks better. The newer *composite resins* (white) can be bonded directly to the enamel, and they are stronger than the older type of white fillings called *silicates*. Composite resins are also being used for back teeth. Eventually, they may make silver fillings obsolete. They cost about the same as a silver filling, so you may prefer them.

The *gold filling* (inlay) is used primarily when the decay is very large and a silver filling would not be strong enough. It requires an impression and it cannot be completed in one visit because it must be fabricated by a laboratory technician. It could cost you five times as much as a silver or white filling. If your dentist suggests a gold inlay, you may decide to spend a little more and have a porcelain jacket crown.

Many prosthetic restorations, like crowns and fixed bridgework, are expensive, and consumers who consider *only* the fee can be making a mistake by choosing cheaper work. Obviously, a lot depends on your budget. On the other hand, you could consider paying off or borrowing for this kind of investment in your dental health. Most consumers don't hesitate to pay off cars, TVs, and furniture. Even vacations which are pure luxury items advertise "Fly Now, Pay Later." Why not "Look and Feel Better Now, Pay Later?" An investment in your health, appearance, and general psychological well being can be the best thing you ever paid off.

PROSTHETIC CONSUMER TIPS

- Don't wait six months after your teeth have been extracted to have full dentures made. Your bone ridge can resorb and your facial features can sag. Consider immediate dentures to eliminate the waiting period. You can have them relined for $50-75 later on.
- Expect a period of adjustment while you get used to the feel of artificial teeth and learn to speak and eat with them.
- Don't expect perfection of false teeth. Be realistic. You can make a reasonable adjustment if you are persistent and you don't expect your false teeth to be as good as your natural teeth.
- Wear your dentures when you go to the dentist for an adjustment. He has to see the irritation spots to correct your plate, so you could be wasting a visit if you "wear" them in your pocket.
- Don't try to make your own adjustments or repairs. Do-it-yourself kits can cause irreparable harm to your mouth tissue, and you can wind up paying double for new plates.
- Don't think your troubles are over once you have false teeth. They may be just beginning. Continue to have checkups as your mouth changes and the dentures wear in.
- Chew slowly, take smaller bites, and divide the food equally on both sides. Experiment cautiously with different foods until you learn the tricks that work for you.
- Avoid extraction mills for cheap assembly line dentures, and avoid dental laboratory technicians who operate illegally.
- Save whatever teeth you have. Replace missing teeth promptly. If you don't, the adjacent teeth will drift and cause you additional expense later on.
- Baking soda is cheaper than denture cleaners and works as well. Soap is also acceptable.
- A partial removable denture costs less than a fixed bridge but has definite disadvantages. So although a fixed bridge costs more initially, it's a superior restoration and a better "buy" in the long run.
- If your dentist suggests a crown for a badly decayed tooth and you can't afford it, ask about a filling with reinforcing pins at a fraction of the cost of a crown.
- For your comfort during extensive grinding, ask for Vaseline for your lips, ear plugs to mask the wizz of the drill, and brief rest periods to close your mouth.

- Don't necessarily turn down superior dentistry that costs more. Consider taking out a loan and paying it off like furniture or a car.
- Don't select stark white teeth. A row of gleaming white chicklets in perfect alignment is a dead giveaway.

EXODONTIA

An exodontist, more accurately called an oral surgeon, specializes in the extraction of teeth as well as surgery of the mouth, jaws, and related structures.* Your own dentist will perform simple extractions. But if you run into a problem like an impacted wisdom tooth, a broken root tip, or a tooth that's been pushed up into the sinus, you will probably be referred to an oral surgeon.

Most people think of the oral surgeon as the specialist who *only* extracts teeth. Actually, he is highly trained to do many more complicated surgical procedures. What are they?

The most common one is the removal of an impacted wisdom tooth (Fig. 8-6) which is pressing against another healthy tooth and causing pain. The impacted wisdom tooth is buried in the bone under the gum, far back in the mouth in a very inaccessible area. The oral surgeon has to make an incision in the gum and flap back the gum tissue. Then a "window" has to be cut in the bone large enough to remove the tooth, much like a "Caesarian section" birth. Sometimes the wisdom tooth has to be sectioned into several pieces while still imbedded in the bone, and then lifted out piece by piece through the "window." If your dentist thinks your 16 year old's wisdom tooth will be impacted, it may be wiser to have it out at 16 than at 30 when it can cause more trouble.

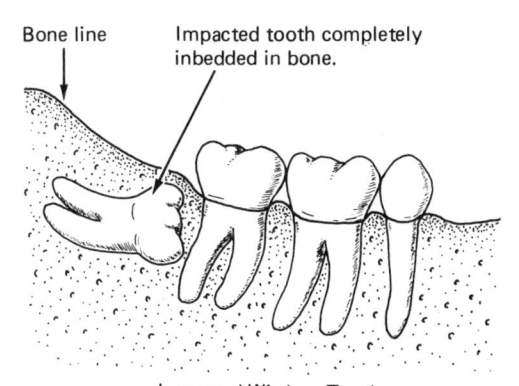

Impacted Wisdom Tooth

Fig. 8-6

*There were 2524 exodontists in 1973, excluding the Armed Forces. Many exodontists prefer the term oral and maxillo-facial surgeon.

If you have a *dental* insurance plan, check to see if you are covered. If you have a *medical* surgical policy, you might be covered for oral surgical procedures such as a biopsy or a fracture. Some insurance policies stipulate that they will only pay for extraction of a wisdom tooth if it is done in a hospital. So even though this *can* be done in the oral surgeon's office, it may be to your advantage to go to the hospital to collect on the policy and save money. Insurance companies should note that when policy coverages are liberalized to allow impacted wisdom teeth and other surgical procedures to be done as an office visit, both the insurance company *and* the patient will save money. Also unnecessary hospital visits will be cut down.

One of the most dramatic oral surgery procedures involves a case in which the patient has a very large pronounced lower jaw that juts out, sometimes called a "lantern jaw" or "bulldog jaw." The oral surgeon may remove a section of the lower jawbone *on each side* and then slide or reposition the lower jaw (mandible) *backward* until a pleasing

Section of lower "LANTERN JAW" removed

BEFORE SURGERY

Jaw repositioned

AFTER SURGERY

Cosmetic Oral Surgery

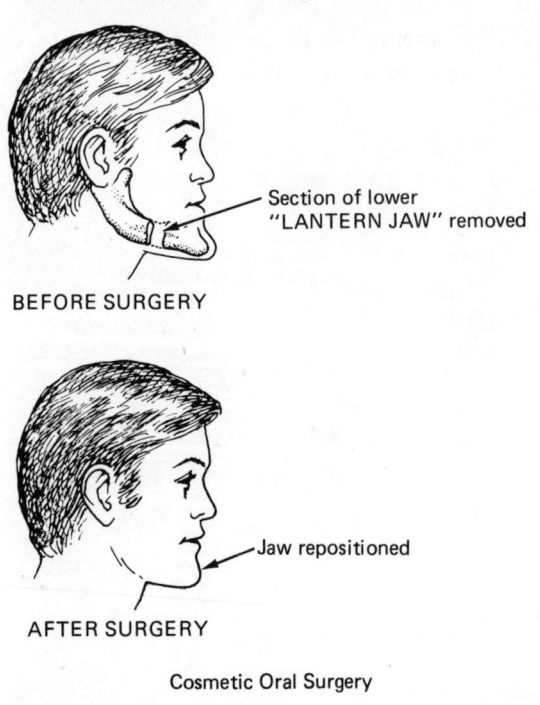

Fig. 8-7

facial harmony is obtained. (Fig. 8-7) This operation is usually done in conjunction with an orthodontist, who helps plan how the teeth will mesh in their new jaw position. The opposite case is the short "Andy Gump" jaw which needs to be lengthened. Here the oral surgeon slides the mandible *forward* to surgically reposition the jaw so it will be more prominent. This type of surgery might be labeled *orthodontic cosmetic surgery,* and the results are nothing short of miraculous. Not only has the patient's bite and appearance been markedly improved, but his personality usually undergoes a terrific boost, too. With increased dental awareness and better insurance coverage, more people are seeking the services of oral surgeons for cosmetic jaw and facial surgery. You don't have to be a television personality like Rona Barrett to be "remade."

The oral surgeon is often called in on an accident case where the patient suffers a fractured jaw as a result of a car smashup, with accompanying lacerations to the lips, cheeks, and tongue, and loosened teeth. If it is a simple fracture, the oral surgeon will wire the upper teeth to the lower teeth to immobilize both jaws for about six weeks. But if the jaw is broken into many fragments, and perhaps sticks through the cheek, the bony pieces have to be reset into position. This is called "reducing the fracture." Facial fractures may require supporting the cheekbones with hooks, pins, or wires.

Another case in which the oral surgeon will be called is when a patient needs a full denture and the ridge of the gums has to be surgically recontoured to accept the plate. Here the oral surgeon will be working with the prosthodontist, who ultimately makes the denture.

Birth defects such as cleft palate (defect in the palate bone) and cleft lip may require the oral surgeon *and* the plastic surgeon to work together *as a team* with the orthodontist, prosthodontist, and speech therapist.

The oral surgeon also treats temporomandibular joint cases, oral cysts, performs surgery of the salivary glands and ducts, and is trained to cope with medical emergencies such as hemorrhage and shock. Patients who have medical complications or are on drugs for medical conditions must be treated with special care. Some heart patients take a blood thinner, some arthritics are on steroid drugs. The oral surgeon is the trained specialist to consult in these cases.

Can these complicated procedures be done in the oral surgeon's office, or is it necessary to go to the hospital? Is it advisable to have general anesthesia whenever an oral surgeon is called in? In many cases, even those as dramatic as setting a broken jaw, the procedures can be done right in the oral surgeon's office and *under local anesthesia.* Remember, local anesthesia is cheaper, less risky, and there is no vomiting or recovery period.

However, some patients fear dental work so much that the *only* way they will submit to it is under general anesthesia. Young children who are hysterical and cannot be reasoned with, disturbed patients, and patients with neuromuscular problems may need a general anesthesia. The oral surgeon is trained to administer general anesthesia to these people. A safe and pleasant way to have oral surgery done in the office is to have a combination of local anesthesia and an intravenous drug administered in such doses as to completely prevent pain *without putting the patient completely to sleep,* a technique called *chemanesia* by Leonard M. Monheim, D.D.S.

If you have decided to have general anesthesia, make sure you know exactly which teeth are going to be extracted *before* you "go to sleep." In rare cases, patients wake up with more teeth out than they bargained for. Have the diagnosis for extraction *made* by your general dentist and *reconfirmed* by the oral surgeon as a second opinion.

After an extraction, take some simple precautions and follow the oral surgeon's instructions (often printed and given to you on leaving his office). Remember, you've had an operation, so give the blood clot time to form, and don't disturb it for a few days. To control bleeding, place a clean gauze pad over the wound and bite down *gently,* maintaining a pressure for about 30 minutes. An ice bag or cold cloth immediately after an extraction can reduce swelling and discomfort. In some cases of tooth extractions, a "dry socket" occurs afterwards. This is a localized inflammation of the empty tooth socket and it can be painful. Call your dentist if pain persists.

What about cancer? The majority of oral cancers are first seen by the dentist. But if you discover *any growth or sore that doesn't heal,* be sure to have your dentist look at it.

> **Dentist Spots Martha Mitchell's Cancer**
>
> *One of the late Martha Mitchell's earliest signs of myeloma, the malignancy that took her life, was first picked up in August, 1975. How? By her dentist, who examined her swollen gums and advised her to see a hematologist immediately. She didn't. In September, despite intense pain in her neck, she refused an X ray and appeared on the Mike Douglas TV show. It was her last public appearance.*

Pipe smokers may discover sores which could develop into cancer. Cheek biters can cause small nodular growths called *polyps* (fibromas) to appear. Some sores heal rapidly and do *not* need to be removed. But any masses or lumps should be examined and watched. If they change, and are suspicious growths, your dentist will decide to have a biopsy done of the tissue to check for malignancy. Malignancies *can* be treated successfully, so don't ignore a growth in the mouth. A prominent New Jersey oral surgeon says, "I've known of growths that were watched and became malignant. If I had a growth, I'd want a microscopic examination of it. It's easy to do!" And don't treat a sore with a mouthwash or gargle with a home remedy. Ask your dentist to diagnose it. If surgery is required, he will send you to an oral surgeon.

Does smoking cause cancer? Most people know smoking increases their risk of developing lung cancer, but they don't know smoking also increases their odds for getting cancer of the mouth and throat. Deaths from this disease are four times higher among smokers than non-smokers. Serious periodontal disease is also increased with smoking. Each year about 7,000 people die of oral cancer, so if you don't smoke, don't start. If you do smoke, stop. If you see any sore on the lips, gums, or inside the mouth that will not heal, any swelling or numbness, or any pain or bleeding, *see your dentist.* Early detection and prompt oral surgery can save your life.

There is another oral surgical procedure that is on the rise, called *implants.* This means the oral surgeon implants a nonreactive metal post or structure into the bone of either the upper or lower jaw where there are teeth missing (if there is enough bone to accommodate the implant). These implants are used in place of natural teeth, and they are becoming more common. If the oral surgeon performs the implant, the general dentist or prosthodontist will build the replacement to fit over the implants.

> **Early Egyptians Tried Dental Implants**
>
> *Dental implantology goes back to the time of the early Egyptians. Mummies and skeletons have been examined, and they indicate that dental implants were attempted even in those days.*

Throughout this book it has been stressed that you should avoid extractions and save your teeth. However, there are certain clear cut indications for extractions. Here are some guidelines you should know.

1. An impacted wisdom tooth that is infected or "leaning" on a sound tooth may cause pain and damage to that tooth and should come out.
2. Extraction of teeth for orthodontic reasons could be necessary when the teeth are so crowded into the jawbone that *only* by removing teeth can room be created to realign the remaining teeth.
3. A tooth that is very loose and mobile is a candidate for extraction. When a tooth can be moved in every direction, including up and down, it can indicate that there is no bone around the root of the tooth. A tooth that is only held in by tissue is a hopeless tooth and cannot be retained.
4. Sometimes a perfectly healthy tooth is extracted solely for cosmetic reasons. A tooth that is out of line and protrudes into the lip may be extracted and replaced with a bridge. The cosmetic improvement can offset the loss of the tooth, which was unsightly and probably harmful to the bite.
5. Unfortunately, some teeth are removed for purely financial reasons. A patient that has a severe toothache in an upper molar with three roots may be faced with the decision of paying $10 for an extraction or $250 for root canal work. The excruciating pain, coupled with his financial pinch, compels him to opt for extraction.

EXODONTIA CONSUMER TIPS

Realistically, the dental consumer who has been referred to an oral surgeon does not have much control over his destiny. You must trust your general dentist's decision to refer you to an oral surgeon, just as you trust your general practitioner to refer you to a heart surgeon. However, there are certain areas of control that you can exercise as a consumer spending money for oral surgery.

- Have the diagnosis for extraction *made* by your general dentist and *reconfirmed* by the oral surgeon. Avoid extraction, unless it is clearly spelled out as the *only* way to achieve the desired result.
- Whenever possible, request *local* anesthesia over *general* anesthesia (going deeply to sleep). Local is safer, painless, and will cost you less money.
- If you will be given a general anesthesia, make sure you and the oral surgeon agree exactly which teeth are to be extracted *before* you go to sleep (so you don't wake up with more teeth extracted than you bargained for).
- Don't neglect any sore or growth in the mouth. Don't treat yourself at home with local mouthwashes. Have your dentist examine the growth for changes, or biopsy the tissue if it seems suspicious.
- Oral cancer deaths are four times higher among smokers than nonsmokers. Early detection and prompt oral surgery could save your life.
- Check your insurance coverage for restrictions of oral surgery. If payments are made *only* if the surgery is performed in a hospital, then have it done there and save the money.
- "Lantern jaws" and "Andy Gump" jaws can be surgically repositioned with miraculous cosmetic and psychological results. Other surgical procedures like cleft palates, recontouring dental ridges, and implants may require the "team" of an oral surgeon, orthodontist, prosthodontist, plastic surgeon, and speech pathologist.

9
How to Get the Most for Your Money by Turning Your Dentist On

Some people prefer to leave everything to their dentist. They believe they can go to him and, presto-chango, all their dental problems will vanish. Although they shop vigorously and knowledgeably for a mechanic to tune up their car engine, or an insurance agent to suggest a homeowner's policy, their consumer awareness stops short of their dentist's waiting room. Why? Because they *do not think of themselves as dental consumers.* They think of themselves as mere patients, and they are content to "turn themselves over" to their dentist. They harbor the mistaken belief that dental care is not their "business." They feel patients should defer to their capital D Dentist who knows best. They say, "He knows what he's doing, I don't," so they rarely ask questions. They are content to rely on sublime faith and confidence in their Dentist, that all knowing, all powerful, all beneficent figure who "will do the right thing."

If you, too, play the role of a humble, submissive patient, there is nothing much you can do to *turn your dentist on.* But if you consider yourself an aware dental consumer, you can exert control to get high quality dentistry, more comfort, and your dental dollars' worth.

First, disregard the mistaken notion that your dentist is some superhuman figure who knows everything about dentistry and always behaves in your highest interests. Even the Greek Gods exhibited remarkably human traits, and like those divine figures your dentist also can behave in remarkably human terms. No one performs at peak efficiency all the time. He can be irritated, tired, even mistaken. He can be generous, brilliant, and charming. He can be charitable or mercenary, considerate or rude, rigid or tolerant, pedantic or homespun. He's human! If you insist on playing the role of *mere patient* to his capital D Dentist, all you can do is submit. But if you're a *wise dental consumer,* you can *turn your dentist on* and consistently reap subtle benefits. Of course, if you've already made the mistake of selecting an incompetent dentist (yes, Virginia, there are incompetent dentists) there's not much you can do except change dentists. But assuming your dentist is reasonably professional (most are), there is latitude for you to work your magic. You can receive better treatment and save some fees on your dental bills. If you learn the knack of *turning your dentist on* to his best performance, you will get those little extra attentions you deserve; some, without paying a dime. You will save time and money and reap fringe benefits you never dreamed of.

For example, you were told at your initial examination you have nine cavities at $10 each. While completing the work, your dentist discovers an additional tiny pit cavity. If you've *turned him on,* he may include the additional work *at no charge* (I have done this countless times). But if you've consistently *turned him off,* he will undoubtedly advise you of the extra procedure and charge you the additional fee (I have done this, too).

This scenario is played out thousands of times in thousands of offices across the country. Why not be the one to save the $10, the time, the extra visit, and the transportation or baby sitting costs? After all, it's your teeth, your dental comfort, and your dental dollars. If we exclude the obviously sleazy or shoddy dental work performed by incompetent or unscrupulous dentists, we will see that there is a considerably wide spectrum of acceptability in dentistry. There is work that is satisfactory, but not exceptional. There is treatment that is acceptable, but not preferential. Many will settle for the satisfactory and acceptable, when they could be getting all the extra benefits of exceptional work and preferential treatment. Why not you? You can *turn your dentist on* and derive real extras in attention and treatment, *many times free of charge.*

There are countless minor office fees you can save that are normally and correctly charged to patients. These fees are due the dentist and he's entitled to charge for them. However, if you learn the ways to *turn your dentist on,* you could find he will waive some of those fees because you are a preferred patient.

For example, Harriet L., a patient of long standing, brought her visiting mother-in-law into my office for relief of a sore spot from the denture made by her dentist in Florida. I had every right to charge for that adjustment. But because Harriet and her family had been considerate patients for many years, I adjusted her mother-in-law's denture, worked her in rapidly between my appointments, and waived the fee.

I am not a saint, nor am I alone in this flexible policy. Many of my colleagues report similar scenarios played out daily in their own offices. They also extend themselves to patients who *turn them on,* those preferred patients who know how to get that little extra from every human contact.

Dr. K, a prominent New York orthodontist, told me of the $50 fee he waived for a preferred patient who had accidentally lost his orthodontic retainer while swimming. Ordinarily, he would have charged $50, even $75, to replace the patient's retainer, and he was entitled to that fee. However, the boy's family had referred numerous friends to him, and in 18 months of treatment the boy had followed instructions to the letter, cutting down on the treatment time. Dr. K. simply waived the fee.

Dr. B. has an office policy of charging $10 for missed appointments. This policy is printed at the bottom of all his bills and he sticks to it as a matter of principle. Nevertheless, in the case of Martin L., who had a spotless record for 16 years, he chose to waive the fee when Martin missed his appointment without calling.

Some dentists adhere to their policies rigidly. They are purists who establish a procedure and a fee and never (or almost never) waver. However, my own experience in interviewing many colleagues is that most dentists are flexible and take into account the situation and past performance record of their patients. Consequently, they react accordingly.

A common situation reported by my colleagues is the patient who returns to the office, complaining bitterly about the filling "you just put in and it fell out." Their attitude is hostile, accusatory, even resentful. They imply that you gypped them, and you'd better do something about it. You check your records and find the filling was done some 10 months ago, and you advise the patient that the tooth must be refilled at a charge of $15. Had that person been a preferred patient whose attitude was different, it is possible the dentist might have waived the charge.

There are many other ways you can save. Perhaps your dentist gives out samples of toothpaste, toothbrushes, or disclosing tablets. This is a common procedure among prevention oriented dentists. Or perhaps your dentist suggests you try a particular over-the-counter dental product or painkiller which he keeps in the office. If you are a preferred patient, he may give you a handful of samples that could save you money at the pharmacy.

Your dentist can instruct his secretary to schedule you so there is little waiting time. A preferred patient who lives or works nearby can receive the extra courtesy in which the dentist has the secretary phone ten minutes before his appointment to "come right over." This is an enormous saving in time and money to a busy executive.

There are other subtle but effective ways to receive preferred treatment. For the patient who *turns him on,* the dentist may make morning appointments when he and his staff are fresh and at their best — when he knows he turns in a peak performance. He can do quadrant dentistry, reducing the chair time to perhaps four visits, where each quadrant is completed at a single sitting. This will not only save you time, but reduce the number of shots necessary to complete the work and thereby reduce your discomfort and stress. He can work with an especially light touch, be extraordinarily considerate of elderly or infirm patients, perhaps even make a house call in rare cases.

If you have learned the knack of *turning your dentist on,* you may find him unusually helpful in preparing an insurance claim worth hundreds, even thousands of dollars. He may advise you how to properly fill out the forms so that you will get all the benefits to which you are entitled. He might read the fine print of your insurance policy and conform the necessary treatment to maximize your benefits, saving you hundreds of dollars. For example, suppose your policy has a maximum coverage of $500 per calendar year and you have $1200 worth of work to be scheduled. He could, perhaps, break up the work into two phases, suggesting half the work be done in one calendar year November to December, and the balance in the next year January to February. This will give you an extra $500 in insurance coverage. A routine patient might have missed this opportunity and had all the work done at once. But a preferred patient would probably get this "extra" attention from his dentist.

If your dentist decides to refer you to a specialist, he might take a little extra time to make the appointment for you instead of leaving it to you. In his conversation with the specialist, he could tip him off that you are "a patient of long standing" or "an old friend," a code to his colleague to extend that extra preferred attention to you.

If you have *turned your dentist on,* he may make an extra effort to come to the telephone when you call him, to be extra patient and communicative when explaining exactly how and why he is performing a particular procedure. He may give you tips which could save you time and money. Everyone likes that little extra bit that translates to V.I.P. treatment. The giftwrapped package is far more attractive than the one in the brown paper bag. You can be the one to derive those extras if you *turn your dentist on.* How? How can you reap the benefits of V.I.P. treatment?

Dentists vary in what turns them on or off. They respond differently to a variety of situations, and their responses vary in intensity. One dentist may fume if his patient is five minutes late, another may enjoy the break. In interviewing many colleagues, the general dentist and the specialist, certain *turn ons* and *turn offs* reappear with a surprising degree of frequency. Here is a representative composite of the common *turn ons* and *turn offs* that *you* can control to get that preferential treatment.

Brush Your Teeth Just Prior to Your Dental Appointment.

This simple courtesy is the most easy, obvious way to *turn your dentist on.* Every dentist appreciates the patient who is thoughtful enough to brush before his visit. I have even observed patients who bring their own toothbrush and toothpaste to my office and go into the lavatory immediately before their appointment. I appreciate that extra consideration. It is easier and more pleasant for a dentist to work in a clean mouth than to spend several minutes flushing and cleaning the food residue from the mouth of a thoughtless patient.

The clod who goes to his dental appointment immediately after eating offensive garlic, onions, or salami is totally inconsiderate of his dentist. Such behavior is inexcusable. The least the patient can do is rinse out his mouth thoroughly with the paper cup *before* the dentist starts. If he insists on presenting a mouth covered with spaghetti sauce and the remains of his antipasto still wedged between his teeth, he can be sure he will be dubbed "the dirty mouth" patient, and he will be given the same degree of consideration he has exhibited. The patient who seats himself in the dental chair chewing gum, or with a candy still in his mouth, is also inconsiderate. The patient smoking a cigarette who blithely asks, "Where can I douse this, Doc?" is killing any chances for special services. He will, in fact, pay for every possible service and get short shrift in the bargain.

Don't go to your dentist immediately after eating, offering up a mouthful of food debris. An apology won't help. Your dentist's irritation at having to spend extra time cleaning up before he starts working will only guarantee you less attention for wasting his time. You have given him the job you should have done yourself, and you'll probably pay for it. A considerate patient would not go to his physician for his annual checkup without bathing and wearing fresh underwear. Don't present a dirty mouth to your dentist. That's a *turn off.*

Be Considerate of Your Dentist's Time.

The major commodities your dentist has to offer are his time and his professional expertise. Your dentist's office is unlike a department store or factory where income and production continues even in the absence of the boss. If your dentist is not working at the chair, he is not producing any income. Consequently, a patient who is consistently late for appointments, misses appointments, or cancels appointments at the last minute, is using up one of the dentist's major commodities without paying for it: Time. Such patients who flout common consideration for their dentist's time may find themselves confronted with definite countermeasures employed to regain that lost income. For example, they may be charged an office fee for a missed appointment. Any patient unwilling to accept that policy may be advised nicely to seek another dentist. Another countermeasure is to keep that patient waiting for weeks, even months, before booking another appointment, or to keep him waiting in the waiting room "to cool his heels." It is certainly to your advantage to observe appointments. This is one way to show you are aware of the value of your dentist's time. Flagrant abuses can only serve to *turn him off.*

You can also be considerate when arranging new appointments with the secretary. The patient who spends five minutes trying to recall if her bridge game was cancelled Tuesday, or wastes time with lengthy, superfluous explanations, is irritating. "Umm, let's see, wasn't I supposed to have my hair done Friday, no that's right I changed it to Saturday for Janie's carpool because my mother-in-law couldn't . . ." That's a time waster. The difficult appointment maker who is so busy he can't come at several suggested times invites uncooperative behavior from the office staff. So does the patient who invariably requires a "special appointment."

"Could you stay a little later for me, Doc?"

"Can't you work me in over the lunch hour?"

"Could you open up a little early so I can get to work?"

These are unreasonable demands that rarely bring forth first class treatment. The patient who can't make it on Saturday morning, is busy Tuesday afternoon, and has a tennis match on Friday, is *not* going to *turn his dentist on.* The message here is that his dental work carries a very low priority, so why should his dentist give him high priority treatment? Of course, most dentists will make a special appointment for a valid reason. But consistently difficult patients will find it equally difficult to get special treatment.

There are other kinds of time wasters who carelessly, perhaps even unknowingly, take small but annoying chunks out of their dentist's time. One is "the rinser." His dentist asks him to rinse, perhaps to wash away a small amount of saliva, blood, or particles of filling. "The rinser" proceeds to use three cups of water, gargling and swishing for several minutes, giving his dentist a slow burn. All that was asked for was a fast swish, then head right back in position. The two minute "rinser" has wasted his dentist's time.

Another is "the wetter." The dentist has just isolated a tooth with cotton rolls, dried the tooth with a short blast of air and is prepared to fill the cavity. Immediately, "the wetter" closes his mouth and wets the area. This, of course, wastes time and the dentist must repeat the whole procedure. Since filling materials should be placed in as dry a field as possible, wetness during the filling process may weaken the material. Your lip movements introducing saliva to the area are directly under your control. So be alert to what your dentist is doing and try to help him. Don't talk or wet your teeth after he has dried them.

Finally, there is the time-wasting antics of "the talker," the obsessive gabber who can't stop. If the dentist asks him politely, "How's the family?" he launches into a five minute soliloquy detailing Lisa's part in the play, Jeff's art prize, and Steven's A in science. Be brief. If your dentist asks you a question, make your point. That five minute soliloquy by "the talker" is time out of his own appointment, causing his dentist to work hurriedly or to shorten his visit. In either case, he is the loser. If you are a talker, you have put your dentist behind in his schedule and added pressure to his day. This can cost you something too, because you have *turned your dentist off.*

Pay Your Bills on Time.

The best dental services are based on a mutual understanding of the fees involved and prompt payment for the professional services you have received. If you and your dentist have spoken honestly and directly about his fees, and you have agreed to have the work done, you should honor that agreement by paying your bills on time. A dentist is not likely to give good treatment to the patient who has treated him badly. Everyone, whether plumber, schoolteacher, or stockbroker, wants to be paid for his work, and dentists are no exception. Patients who run up bills, then pay late or ignore those bills, cost the dentist extra time and effort for collection work. This translates to additional money he must spend. Phone calls, dunning notices, and collection agencies add to the costs of running his practice. Consequently, late payers incur his righteous indignation. They *turn him off.* Inevitably, this is reflected in higher fees to you. Recently, some dentists and physicians have posted signs in their waiting rooms.

> DUE TO THE INCREASED COST OF BILLING, PATIENTS ARE REQUESTED TO PAY FOR EACH OFFICE VISIT BEFORE LEAVING. PLEASE HELP US KEEP FEES DOWN.

There are two distinct aspects to practicing dentistry. One is the scientific part, the treatment of your teeth; the other is the business part, the exchange of money. The dentist in private practice is subject to all the economic pressures of any other business. His dental practice is a business entity governed by the economy, the marketplace, and the spiraling cost of materials and salaries. In order to avail himself of modern equipment, take advanced courses, and maintain a competent staff, he must pay keen attention to the business side of his practice — what business people call "the bottom line." Although dentistry is a healing art, your dentist, like everyone else, is motivated by the profit system, and he wants to be paid for his services. Dentists are not any more or less charitable or mercenary than shopkeepers, and the saying "money talks" is equally applicable to them. Let your money talk by prompt payment of your debts. That's a strong *turn on* to your dentist. It says you value his services and appreciate what he's done.

Of course, partial or delayed payments can be acceptable, too, but don't allow extensive work to proceed if you can't possibly pay for it. Your dentist will probably extend himself to help you find an alternate plan if you are honest at the outset.

A frank discussion *before the work starts* can uncover a mutually acceptable payment plan that is not a burden to you. A six month installment plan, a delayed work plan, or a stopgap plan are all methods to explore directly and openly with your dentist. These will allow you to hold your head high and pay your bills on time. Failure to meet your financial obligations inevitably results in bad feelings, higher costs, and interrupted or incompleted treatments. "Deadbeats," patients who "stick" their dentist, are turned over for collection. Legal action, the last resort, can result in a marred credit rating, court costs, and legal fees. Pay your bills on time and *turn your denitst on.*

Be Pleasant and Cooperative with your Dentist's Staff.

The dental assistant, secretary, and oral hygienist are employed by your dentist to help him give you better and faster treatment. They are, therefore, in a position to give or deny you special attention — those little "extras" that mean so much. If a patient is rude and demanding, he can expect to pay for it in subtle ways. The appointment secretary, for example, may find it "impossible" to fit him in at the time he wants. She may be equally rigid about collecting the bill. There are countless V.I.P. treatments she can offer the "nice" patient: a smile to allay his fears; a cup of coffee; perhaps, a phone call to say his appointment will be delayed.

Most offices, whether they have one assistant, or half a dozen, operate as small cooperative units. Each assistant's job is to help make that office run more smoothly. Unlike employees housed in the steel skyscrapers of a large corporation, dental assistants see each other every day in the same office. They may also have lunch together and belong to the same bowling league or "Y." If a patient is rude to one assistant, she's likely to "tip off" the others. In fact, busy dentists often rely on their assistants for such "tip offs." A word from his assistant that Mrs. Hawkins insulted her will *not* endear Mrs. Hawkins to her dentist. It will *turn him off.* The assistant can predispose or color the relationship between you and your dentist, so don't stack the cards against yourself.

The patient whose attitude is "only the dentist counts," is mistaken. Assistants are an extension of the dentist, and he cannot work smoothly without them. They contribute to his well being and to yours, too. Treat your dentist's staff kindly and you will *turn your dentist on.*

Don't be an Office Nuisance.

Your own home or business follows the particular routine you have established because you feel most comfortable with it. It "works" for you, and it's upsetting when that routine is disturbed. Like you, your dentist has set up his office with the particular routine that serves him best. Consequently, patients who upset it *turn him off.*

Every dental office has simple rules that keep things humming. Perhaps your dentist, like many other preventive-oriented professionals, has placed a sign in his waiting room.

> FOR THE SAKE OF YOUR HEALTH
> AND THE COMFORT OF OTHERS,
> PLEASE DO NOT SMOKE.

A confirmed smoker who is nervous about his visit "needs" a few puffs, so he lights up to the discomfort of everyone else in the waiting room. That's a *turn off.*

Another office nuisance is the person who ties up his dentist's phone with incoming or outgoing calls. "I just have to call my agent," the aspiring actor says, then asks for pencil and paper to list his messages. A worried mother just has to "check with my neighbor to see if Mark got home from school." Another patient receives the inevitable phone call from his wife to "pick up milk and stop at the bakery on your way home." The dental office is *not* the place to transact business.

A few patients, perhaps unwittingly, *turn their dentists off* with gratuitous "dentist jokes" they probably consider witty. "No offense, Doctor, but I hate dentists." (Imagine how you'd feel if your dentist's rejoinder was, "No offense, but I hate patients.") The oldest one is that tired line, "I'd rather have a baby than have a tooth filled." These corny jokes are stale to the dentist, who has heard them dozens of times.

Office nuisances who "take over" the waiting room are a particular thorn to the receptionist. These people sit by idly while their children annoy everyone else waiting. They allow their children to do things they would never permit in their own homes — tear up magazines, run and yell, pound furniture with plastic toys. They turn the waiting room into a luncheonette, leaving a trail of cracker crumbs and jelly smudges.

Don't be an office nuisance.

Dress Appropriately for a Dental Appointment.

Casual clothes are certainly the fashion of today for many occasions that used to call for more formal dress. Restaurants and theaters have relaxed their dress codes for the more appropriate and popular styles, so there is plenty to choose from when going to your dentist.

Patients who wear expensive, dry clean only fabrics put added demands on the dentist. Of course he takes every precaution not to soil your clothing, but rinsing and spitting and spraying can cause a mishap, even with a bib or protective apron covering you.

Men who wear white turtleneck shirts or costly silk ties and expensive suits do not help their dentist by adding anxiety to "look out" for their clothing. Women who come in provocative attire, scanty shorts and halters, and heavy makeup are also inappropriate. "I just had my hair done, so don't mess it.", is a *turn off.* Dangling earrings, thick lipstick, and long false eyelashes only get in the way.

You can help your dentist by dressing appropriately.

Don't be a Hostile, Suspicious Patient.

Dentists, like mothers-in-law, have been stereotyped for years on television, in the movies, and in the comics. Any comedian knows he can count on a "dentist joke" to get a laugh. So it's not surprising that many patients associate dentists with pain. Their reaction, of course, is fear. The two strongest fears associated with dentists are fear of pain and fear of high bills. Some patients, accepting the stereotype of the sadistic dentist out to fleece every patient, have set up negative attitudes that explode the minute they enter the dentist's office. They are openly hostile. They are accusatory. Result? They immediately *turn their dentist off.*

These patients are suspicious of everything. They question the dentist's motives and imply he is exaggerating the amount of work they need to "build up" their case. They are intent on giving their dentist a hard time. They zealously check every procedure and fee. They are convinced they will be overcharged, so they give him the third degree. Such behavior inevitably *turns the dentist off.* The general dentist may "refer out" that kind of patient to get rid of him, send him to a specialist whose fee may run $75 for the initial workup.

Emily J., a 41 year old computer analyst with twenty years experience as a "dentist-hopper," complained bitterly to her dentist. "I've had terrible experiences with every dentist I ever went to," she stated with undisguised suspicion. And Arnold F., a young, newly graduated C.P.A., warned his dentist, "I sued my last dentist and won a nice, fat settlement, Doc, so you better watch your step." He has declared war! It's unlikely that either patient will develop new patterns with their dentists because their hostility undermines any decent relationship. Both patients have *turned their dentist off.*

Don't antagonize your dentist by playing the know-it-all. It's one thing to be an informed consumer, and another to play amateur dentist. The authoritative patient who declares, "Look, Doctor, my sister had the *exact* same thing done and her dentist charged $25 less than you. *He* says . . . ," is only inciting bad feelings. Questioning your dentist in a friendly and informed manner will win his respect. But threatening remarks win contempt which you will pay for. Don't *turn your dentist off* with snide remarks. Don't blame him for past dental experiences. Remember just as you are judging his "chairside manner," he is taking stock of your "patientside manner." Hostility is counterproductive and will bring you a perfunctory, hurried service. In fact, most dentists are likely to "weed out" hostile patients.

Communicate your Symptoms Clearly.

All medical and dental treatments are based on the proper diagnosis of the patient's problem. One of the tools your dentist has to arrive at a correct diagnosis is the information you provide. So be direct and clear in what you report, and weigh your answers to his questions: "Where does it hurt?" "How long has it been bothering you?" "What brings on the pain?" "Does hot or cold intensify it?" "Does it wake you up at night?" "Does the pain radiate anyplace?" "Did you have any swelling?" Try to be alert and observant about changes in your health. If your dentist asks you, "When did that sore first appear on the inside of your cheek?", don't answer with a maddeningly vague, "Gee, maybe last week, I guess, or maybe last month, I'm not sure." Of course, your dentist has scientific diagnostic tools to help him pin down the problem – pulp testers, X rays, his physical examination of your mouth – but you as the patient can offer the most useful, first hand information, if you can communicate your symptoms clearly. On the other hand, unobservant, uncommunicative patients can delay proper diagnosis and treatment by giving their dentist false and vague symptoms.

It helps considerably if you are acquainted with dental procedures and have acquired some basic understanding of dental terminology. It's easier for your dentist to communicate with an informed patient. If he suggests periodontal treatments and you don't know what the words mean, you're at a disadvantage. Some patients are too embarrassed to ask and they proceed through an entire conversation full of explanations that simply "go over their heads." Therefore, they cannot make an informed, knowledgeable decision.

Being an informed consumer carries certain obligations to keep up with the medical-dental advancements that are proliferating — newer treatments, better ways to protect your health, breakthroughs and developments in health care. If you are reading this book, you are already on your way to becoming an informed consumer. You can obtain a lot of *free information* at your dentist's office, from government agencies, at your library, hospital, or public health clinic. Or you can write directly to the:

>   *American Dental Association*
>   *211 East Chicago Street*
>   *Chicago, Illinois 60611*

Ask for their patient education brochures. An informed and communicative patient is a pleasure to your dentist. Communicate clearly and get better treatment. *Turn your dentist on.*

Don't ask your Dentist to Cheat for you.

Patients who carry dental insurance plans sometimes ask their dentist to "put me down for an extra hundred, Doc, because they're going to deduct from my coverage anyhow." They look upon this as a common courtesy due them, and they expect their dentist to "play along because everyone does it." These same people boast of having had identical experiences with "upping" insurance claims on their automobile repairs or their household damages, so they see nothing wrong in asking their dentist to, "Stretch it, Doc, so I don't lose my deductible."

Of course, your dentist has latitude in helping to see that you get every benefit due you, according to the terms of your policy. And there are ways to report the same claim, which can help or hinder you in receiving your fullest benefits. As dental insurance plans cover more and more people, dentists themselves have become more familiar with the forms, and knowledgeable about how to fill them out. Read your own policy first, then bring it with you so your dentist can read it, too. Then ask him to write up the form to maximize your benefits in a perfectly legitimate way. He will try to fit each and every benefit allowed into your treatment plan.

But don't ask him to *lie* for you, to backdate a claim, to state you had more expensive or different treatment from what he actually performed. His professional reputation is at stake, and his dental license can be revoked. You are asking him to sign his name to a fraudulent document, to falsify records and lay his professional career on the line for you. You have *turned him off.*

Compliment your Dentist and be a Booster.

Everyone likes to be told he did a good job, to feel appreciated, and to receive compliments. Compliments nourish the receiver. Parents use compliments effectively in bringing up their children; teachers employ compliments to reinforce learning; and behavior modification therapists apply compliments to encourage particular patterns of behavior. We know that consistent and sincere praise may cause an unpleasant relationship to take an upswing, and motivate people to repeat the approved behavior. If you've been told, "You did a terrific job fixing the stereo," or "Your Thanksgiving dinner was delicious," you will probably "knock yourself out" to perform at that peak again. It feels good to be appreciated.

Dentists who hear complaints all day are especially grateful for the patients who take the time to compliment them when they are pleased. It is a welcome change to receive a compliment instead of a complaint. So let your dentist know. Tell him, "I can eat fine on that side since you fixed the tooth," or "the pain's all gone just like you said," or "it feels perfect, Doctor, and the sore spots disappeared." To the dentist barraged with the unending artillery fire of complaints — "it hurts here"; "my gums are sore"; "they're bleeding and swollen" — it's a special pleasure to hear a compliment. Tell him you feel better, look more attractive, and you appreciate the improvement. Some patients who have established a warm personal relationship of many years with the dental assistants or the dentist say "thank you" with a small gift or a batch of home baked cookies. However you show it, you can *turn your dentist on* by telling him that you appreciate what he's done for you.

The highest compliment you can pay your dentist is to refer a relative, co-worker, or friend to him. It expresses your confidence in him and demonstrates that you appreciate his professional care. When you recommend another person to your dentist, you are letting him know how highly you regard him, and you are helping to expand his practice. You are his booster. This is the ultimate *turn on!*

If you care about getting the most from your dental dollars, you will develop your skills to *turn your dentist on.* Everyone wants to receive the extra bonuses and dividends that elude the ordinary consumer. For a dental consumer, that begins with awareness. The keen observer will notice that his dentist is not only a professional dispenser of health care, but also a skilled craftsman who is performing precision work in a small inaccessible area. His work may be compared to that of a fine jeweler or watchmaker who also does precision work. Except there is *one major difference.* The dentist is working on *you.* A human being is at the end of the drill, not an inanimate object. So he must concentrate on the accuracy of the work as well as be conscious of his chairside manner. He is performing this precision work in a wet field (saliva) and must contend with the movements of your tongue. He is working with powerful, high speed drills where a wrong movement can cause serious damage. He is peering into a mouth mirror which fogs up each time you exhale. When his hand and instrument move to the right, the image in the mirror moves to the left. These are the conditions under which he works every day. And he must adjust to each patient who feels his or her problem is the most pressing. To compound these pressures by *turning your dentist off* can only short change you.

Pressures Mount on Dentists

Dentists have a suicide rate twice as high as that of the U.S. male population. Why? Some explanations may be the pressures and psychological stress associated with their work — the demand for precision in inaccessible areas of the mouth. Tight appointment schedules, compulsive attention to detail, and peer rivalry can be other contributing causes for this statistic.

In Chapter 2 you learned you were entitled to certain definite services from your dentist. In Chapter 3 you did a checkup on your dentist. Now that you have rated him, do you dare to rate yourself? Your spouse? Your children? What kind of patient are you? Do you *turn your dentist on or off?* Take this PATIENT PROFILE test and find out how you rate.

	PATIENT PROFILE	
YOU ARE	DESCRIPTION	SCORE
The DIRTY MOUTH	You eat just before seeing your dentist and don't brush. Food particles are lodged around your teeth.	-2
The APPOINTMENT BREAKER	You are habitually late, don't show up, or cancel the same day.	-3
The LATE PAYER	You are constantly behind in your payments. You make no effort to explain or arrange partial payments.	-3
The RINSER	Your dentist asks you to rinse. He wants a fast swish, you give him a two minute gargle.	-1
The WETTER	Your dentist dries your teeth to work on them. You immediately close your mouth and wet them.	-1
The HOSTILE PATIENT	You complain about every bad dental experience you ever had. You blame your dentist and you're sure he's going to cheat you.	-2
The OFFICE WRECKER	You let your children wreck the waiting room, then reward them with crackers and jelly.	-1
The COMPULSIVE TALKER	Your dentist asks a simple question. You give him a detailed 5 minute soliloquy.	-1
The SPECIAL APPOINTMENT	You insist your dentist stay late for you, open early, or work over his lunch hour.	-1
The TELEPHONE PEST	You have to make an important call and tie up his line.	-1
The FASHION PLATE	You come "dressed to kill," or wear heavy makeup and jewelry.	-1

YOU ARE	DESCRIPTION	SCORE
The NUISANCE	You enter the treatment room with gum, candy, or a cigarette.	-1
The INSURANCE CHEAT	You ask your dentist for a phony statement to collect fraudulent benefits.	-2
The COMMUNICATOR	You are observant and communicate your symptoms clearly and accurately.	+2
The COMPLIMENTER	You are pleased with your dentist and compliment him so he knows he's appreciated.	+2
The BOOSTER	You refer friends and relatives to him, paying him the ultimate compliment.	+3

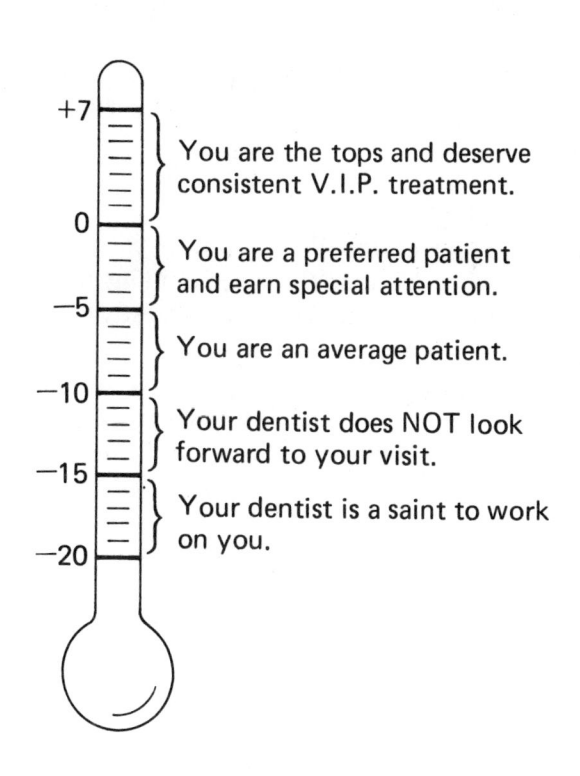

+7 } You are the tops and deserve consistent V.I.P. treatment.

0 } You are a preferred patient and earn special attention.

−5

} You are an average patient.

−10

} Your dentist does NOT look forward to your visit.

−15

} Your dentist is a saint to work on you.

−20

10

When Money's No Object and You Want to Go First Class:
Dentistry for the Rich and the Super Rich

Bryce and Mary Robertson* live on a five acre estate in affluent Short Hills, New Jersey. The approach to their brick Georgian is heralded by a graceful, circular, white pebbled driveway that sweeps past manicured lawns and carefully pruned shrubs, a clay tennis court, and a heated in-ground pool. Parked in front of their three car garage are a shiny black Mercedes Benz, a sparkling white Lincoln Continental, and a sporty red Fiat. The Bryce Robertsons are not Rockefellers or Morgans. But they are rich — very rich.

Bryce Robertson, 52, is an attorney-entrepreneur and senior partner of Robertson, Dickerson, and Holmes, a prestigious Wall Street law firm with 28 junior associates. R.D. & H. represents some of the largest multi-national corporations. Therefore, Bryce Robertson makes frequent business trips to Tokyo, London, and Rome. Transatlantic telephone calls, chauffeured limousines, and private jets are a routine part of his business schedule. His earnings run well into six figures.

Mary Robertson, 49, a couturier dressed, and coiffured suburban matron, is active in her country club, supports charity fund raising affairs, and is an impeccable hostess. With the help of a full time couple, Rose, the maid, and Edward, the gardener-chauffeur, she runs the Robertson family. Mary Robertson has always enjoyed the best in cars, clothes, and country clubs.

Bryce Robertson, Jr., 18, is a Princeton freshman. His sister Jean, 16, is a sophomore at Gil St. Bernard, a private school. Jean boards

*All names are fictitious.

her horse "Sinclair" at a riding stable nearby, and looks after her brother's dalmatian since he left for college.

Six months ago, Bryce Robertson suffered a mild coronary attack. This prompted him to "slow down," and he decided to take better care of himself. Reluctantly, he began to delegate more work to his subordinates. He also acknowledged the fact that he was 25 pounds overweight, smoked too many cigars, and had a receding hairline. To add to his frustrations, his Wednesday tennis game was off and his teeth were bothering him.

Since Robertson was highly skilled at solving problems for his clients, it was an easy shift to harness these same energies to shed 25 pounds, stop smoking, and be fitted for a $500 hair piece that defied detection. The tennis pro at the Club sharpened up his game. Along with all these steps for self-improvement, B. R. decided to find the best dentist around, and put his teeth in perfect shape.

In past years, the law firm had usurped B. R.'s time to such an extent, he could only grudgingly fit in an occasional dental checkup. In fact, his family dentist had warned him five years back that without major dental work, he would lose his teeth. B. R. checked with his family dentist, and was recommended to Dr. Walter White.*

"He's got an outstanding reputation for complete mouth rehabilitation work. He lectures all over the world, he's published articles in the top journals, and he teaches graduate courses in prosthodontia at the dental school. He's damn good. But he's *very* expensive."

"That's okay," B. R. replied. "I want the best!"

"He even has movie stars fly east for his dental miracles."

"Call him and make the appointment!"

Dr. Walter White occupied a seventeen room dental suite in a prestigious building, high above Central Park South. The suite was shared jointly by a periodontist, an endodontist, a young associate, and a staff of ten auxiliaries to assist them. Dr. White accepted only 20 major dental rehabilitation cases per year. The average fee ran over $10,000. Even so, it was not easy to get an appointment. Dr. White's patients had two things in common. They wanted the very best in dentistry; and they were all members of a "club": *the super rich.*

*Fictitious.

Bryce Robertson's secretary confirmed the initial dental appointment for him. On the phone, she was advised that the initial examination and dental evaluation was $200, payable at the conclusion of that visit.

At B. R.'s first visit, he was greeted by the receptionist who asked him to complete a detailed medical-dental history form. Ten minutes later, a dental assistant seated him in a cheerful yellow operatory and made him comfortable. In a moment Dr. White entered, accompanied by his young associate. Several minutes of social pleasantries were exchanged as doctor and patient sized each other up carefully.

"My associate, Dr. Gordon, will take some intra-oral photographs and some impressions for study models," Dr. White explained. "Then Julie, our oral hygienist, will give you an initial cleaning and take a full set of X rays, including our special Panorex film. These preliminary diagnostic tests should take us about an hour and a half," Dr. White concluded. "Then at the next visit, when we have all the diagnostic tests in, we'll have a consultation and lay out some possible treatment plans. How does that sound?"

"Fine. I'm all ready!" B. R. was pleased.

Two weeks later, he returned for his consultation. He waited less than five minutes in the reception center.

Dr. White's examination was thorough and efficient. First, he listened attentively to all B. R.'s dental complaints, his fears, and his expectations. Then he methodically examined each tooth for mobility, sensitivity, and pocket depth with an air blast and a probe. He checked the soft tissues, the cheeks, the tongue, and the floor of the mouth. He checked his patient's bite and examined his jaw movements, his smile, his facial features, and he palpated his temporomandibular joint. Dr. White repeatedly referred to the X rays and study models, as he called out detailed notes to his dental assistant who recorded everything on the dental chart.

"Look, Mr. Robertson, you've neglected your teeth for too long, and it looks like you have a case of advanced periodontal disease."

"I know I've neglected them, Doctor. My dentist warned me about it five years ago, but I was tied up with business obligations and never got to it."

"It's an old story, isn't it? I hear it all the time."

"Can you save my teeth, Doctor? I'll do anything you say, but I don't want to end up with dentures."

"Let me explain this to you. Before we can start any restorative work, you'll have to have some gum surgery. We've got to minimize the pocket depths that exist around your teeth. That means recontouring the gums and the bone; perhaps even a plug of bone."

"Bone transplants?"

"Yes. We take a plug of bone from a healthy section and transplant it into an area that's deficient."

"That's amazing, Doctor."

Dr. White laughed. "Dentistry is not just filling teeth and extracting them. We've come a long way. You see, we can't build bridges on a shaky foundation."

"Of course, just what my dentist told me in New Jersey. He warned me about that five years ago."

"Besides the gum surgery, you'll need root canal therapy on at least three key teeth. Maybe more. Two of the key teeth are in such bad shape that our endodontist will have to remove the weakest root and leave only the strongest."

"Then I won't lose those teeth?"

"No, we can save them with root canal therapy and internal posts."

"Internal posts? What does that mean? Does it hurt?"

"No, no, it won't cause you any pain. Actually, it's quite routine for us. Look, you can do miracles in the courtroom. We do miracles in the mouth."

Bryce Robertson smiled. He liked a professional man who appreciated his own brand of professionalism. He had confidence in Dr. White.

"An internal post is simply a precision gold post that fits up into the root canal to strengthen and support the tooth."

"It's sort of an artificial root to save the tooth. Right?"

"You can think of it that way. However, in addition to this, I'm suggesting a metal implant into your upper jaw bone for additional anchorage to help stabilize the bridgework. I know this all sounds pretty rugged, but believe me, it's painless, and you stand a pretty good chance to save your remaining teeth."

"A metal implant into my jaw bone? How does that work?"

"We part the gum and flap it back. Then we channel a thin groove into the bone. We place a vitallium implant blade into that groove and then gently tap it into place."

"But what holds it into the bone?" B. R. asked. "What keeps it there?"

"The blade is shaped like an ax. Ever split logs? The ax blade is shaped like a wedge, so when you hit bone, it lodges right in there. It's very stable. Another thing: the vitallium blade has holes in it like swiss cheese. And nature does some remarkable things. Your own healthy bone will fill in all those holes."

"You mean my bone grows right into that vitallium blade?"

"Exactly. So the blade becomes anchored to the bone and serves as an extra tooth where your tooth is missing. That blade has a stub sticking up through your gum. And we simply put a crown over it and attach it to the rest of your bridgework. Here, take a look at this." Dr. White showed B. R. an illustration. (Fig. 10-1) "See?"

"That's absolutely amazing. What are the odds that it all works out? It sounds like a lot of work."

"There are no guarantees, but I'll do the best I can. Your work could last only a year or two. But on the other hand, if you practice excellent dental hygiene, it could last the rest of your life."

Bryce Robertson was a man used to making decisions. "Then it's mouth rehabilitation or losing my teeth — eventually wearing dentures. Let's do it! How long will it take?"

"I'd estimate somewhere around seven to nine months. I'd like to see you for a full morning about twice a month. We'd set up a schedule on it."

"And what would the total fee be?"

"I'll prepare a complete and detailed estimate for you. But a ballpark figure would be somewhere between $13,000 and $14,000."

Bryce Robertson did not flinch. He was a man accustomed to fast, accurate judgments; ones which often involved large figures. Also, he had been alerted by his family dentist to expect the fee to fall in that range, and recently had instituted a Delta Insurance Plan for all key personnel at Robertson, Dickerson, and Holmes. It covered him to $1000 a year. Furthermore, he quickly calculated that it would be no financial strain. Since his annual income was well over $100,000, in his tax bracket the dental fee would substantially lower his income

DENTISTRY FOR THE RICH AND THE SUPER RICH   215

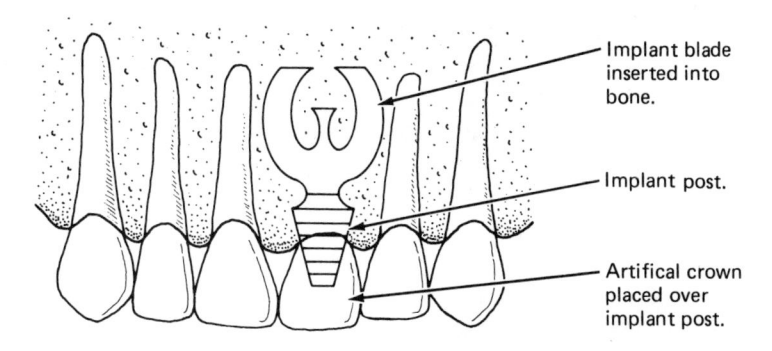

Implant blade inserted into bone.

Implant post.

Artifical crown placed over implant post.

Single tooth Replacement with an Implant.

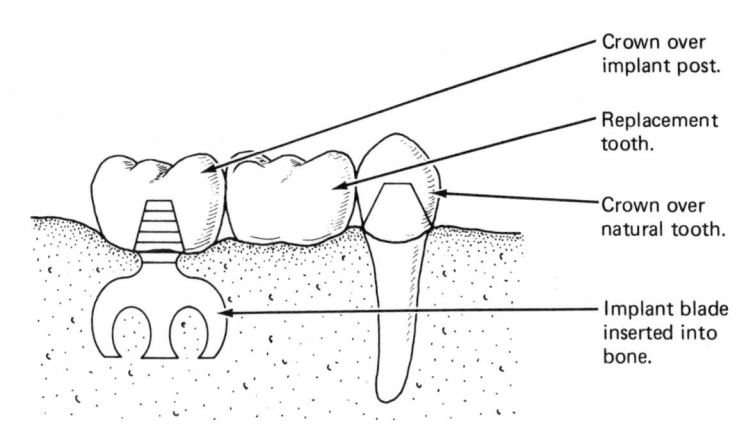

Crown over implant post.

Replacement tooth.

Crown over natural tooth.

Implant blade inserted into bone.

Implant used as an "Anchor" for a Fixed Bridge.

Fig. 10-1

tax. Better to spend it on a stunning new smile for Bryce Robertson, he thought, than give it to Uncle Sam. Psychologically, emotionally, and financially he was ready. He didn't want to lose his teeth, his vitality, or his sex appeal. He didn't want to feel old.

"When do we start?" he snapped back with confidence.

Nine months later, Bryce Robertson sported the best that dentistry had to offer: A Hollywood smile of 28 shiny, porcelain jacket crowns. He felt ten years younger and couldn't wait to get back on the tennis courts.

Here's what he got for his money.

Walter White, D.D.S.
Central Park South
New York City

Treatment Plan and Estimate for Bryce Robertson, Short Hills, New Jersey.

Initial Examination, photographs, study models, X-rays, prophylaxis, and diagnosis	$200.
Periodontal surgery, four quadrants, including gingivoplasty and osteoplasty.	$2,400.
Root Canal Therapy of 3 molar teeth, root resection of 2 teeth	$900.
Vitallium implant	$500.
28 units, porcelain crowns.	$10,000.
TOTAL FEE	$14,000.

Bryce Robertson filed this away to present to his tax accountants, so he could take the proper deductions on his substanital income tax.

(Mary R.) Unlike her husband, Mary Robertson had always taken meticulous care of her teeth. Although she was not endowed with particularly trouble-free teeth, she more than compensated by exercising fastidious oral hygiene. She was compulsive and methodical about seeing her dentist every three months for a prophylaxis and checkup.

About eight years ago, Mary R. had extensive periodontal surgery, with multiple crowns of gold with plastic veneers. She was now concerned with the way the plastic facings of these crowns had gradually discolored, causing a rim of gold on the gum line to show up as an unsightly dark line. Her dentist reassured her that the crowns were still functionally perfect, and the rim of gold along the gum line was caused by some recession of her gums.

Nevertheless, this cosmetic imperfection was a source of some displeasure to her, and she convinced her dentist to remake the crowns for purely aesthetic reasons. She wanted to look better. Her husband also encouraged her to redo her mouth.

"It makes sense," he explained, "from an income tax point of view, to lump all our dental expenses together in one fiscal year. Besides, Mary, my dental insurance plan covers you, too. That's another $1000, so let's use it!"

Mary Robertson made arrangements to have her six crowns remade at a cost of $300 per unit. Total: $1800. Her dentist reemphasized that these new crowns were being made for strictly cosmetic reasons, since the old crowns were still adequate from a functional point of view. This time, however, her crowns would be constructed from porcelain fused to gold.

"Unlike the plastic veneers, this type of crown won't discolor over the years," her dentist said.

Mary Robertson's dental bill for the year was just under $2000, which included six porcelain crowns, X rays, prophylaxis, and minor routine care.

(Bryce Jr.) The Robertson children also had been given the very best in dental health care. They were fed fluoride vitamins from birth, and their pedodontist insisted on topical fluoride treatments at each six month checkup. They also used fluoride toothpaste exclusively, since the water in Short Hills was not fluoridated. Mary saw, too, that her children established good, nutritious dietary habits, although Bryce Jr. admitted he had slipped a bit, since dormitory life at Princeton encouraged munching junk food. Nevertheless, this early regime of dental care and good habits of hygiene proved effective, because Bryce Jr. and his sister Jean both had a low incidence of caries over their school years.

Bryce Jr. had a beautiful smile. He was able to avert orthodontic treatment because his pedodontist had wisely inserted a space maintainer to guide his permanent teeth into proper occlusion. This interceptive orthodontic appliance was made when Bryce was 8, and it probably eliminated long and costly orthodontic treatments at 14.

"When all the other guys were "Brace Faces" in ninth grade, I had straight teeth and smiled a lot to show them off," he admitted.

Two years ago, when Bryce Jr. chipped two front teeth in a basketball game, his parents were concerned that he would need crowns to restore his appearance. But their dentist suggested that the chipped corners of the teeth could be restored with *composite resins,* eliminating the need for costlier crowns.

"What does that mean, Doctor?" Mary asked.

"A composite resin is a filling material the color of natural teeth. It bonds and adheres directly to the tooth surface, and we match the color exactly. It's a relatively new material in dentistry, and it's superior to the older porcelain filling materials because it bonds and we don't have to drill. It'll be perfect for Bryce Jr.'s front teeth."*

Mary R. was pleased. She knew two crowns would run about $600. The *composite resin restorations* would cost only $60. She prided herself on being a "good manager" and a knowledgeable consumer.

"Then a composite resin isn't silver like an amalgam filling. And it's better than the porcelain fillings you usually use on front teeth, because it sticks to the tooth without drilling."

"Bryce Jr.'s two front teeth will look just like his own teeth looked before the accident," her dentist assured her. "As a matter of fact, see that space between his two front teeth? We can repair that space — we call it a *diastema* — exactly the same way with a composite resin restoration."

He drew Mary and Bryce Jr. a picture (Fig. 10-2) and they immediately agreed to repair the two teeth cosmetically with composite resins.

"I think I'll come out ahead on this accident," Bryce Jr. told his mother. "You know, that space between my teeth used to bother me, but I figured I couldn't do anything about it. This sounds really simple."

Diastema Doesn't Mar Model

Top cosmetic model Lauren Hutton pulls a $200,000 a year salary for her smile which includes a prominent and uncorrected diastema. Apparently, "the rows of pearls" look is a thing of the past. Look where the "gap" got her.

Recently, however, Bryce Jr. ran into another problem — impacted wisdom teeth. His gums in the back of his mouth were sore and

---

*If you are having fillings done on your front teeth, ask your dentist if they are *composite resins.* If you've chipped a tooth, maybe you don't need a crown. Ask if a composite resin will do the job.

DENTISTRY FOR THE RICH AND THE SUPER RICH 219

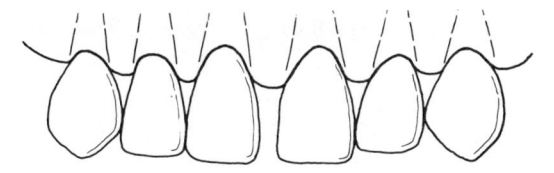

A. Indicates the way Bryce Robertson, Jr. looked **BEFORE** he chipped his two front teeth. Note the "Diastema" or space between the front teeth.

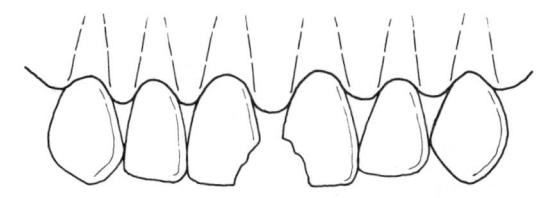

B. Indicates the way he looked **AFTER** his teeth were chipped.

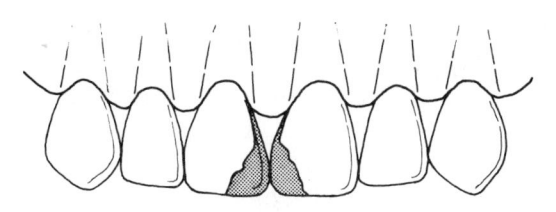

C. Restorations with **COMPOSITE RESINS** corrected both the fractured teeth and eliminated the "Diastema". Shaded areas of composite resins match color of natural teeth.

Fig. 10-2

painful, and he even had shooting pains into his ear. His dentist referred him to an oral surgeon, and he had all four impacted wisdom teeth removed during spring vacation. Cost? $500.

(Jean) Jean Robertson, now a sixteen year old high school student, had crowded buck teeth when she was in Junior High, two and a half

years back. At that time she had four teeth extracted, because her orthodontist felt her jaw was too small to fit all her teeth into proper position. Mary Robertson secured the "top" specialist in the area to do Jean's orthodontic work. His fee (a "top" fee for two and a half years of treatment) was $2400. Of this, $500 was covered by Jean's father's dental insurance.

Jean's orthodontist used the new clear plastic brackets, which bond directly to teeth, instead of unsightly metal bands. Jean was a cooperative patient like her mother and kept all her appointments, so her orthodontic work went smoothly and gave excellent results. Now Jean wears a retainer to keep her teeth from drifting back. She is thrilled that her teeth are straight, and she can go off to college with a beautiful smile.

What did the Robertson family spend on their mouths? Here's what the total picture added up to.

ROBERTSON FAMILY DENTAL DOLLARS SCOREBOARD

Bryce Robertson	complete mouth rehabilitation	$14,000.
Mary Robertson	cosmetic dentistry (6 crowns)	2,000.
Bryce Jr.	oral surgery (4 impactions)	500.
Jean	orthodontic treatments (spread over 2 ½ years)	2,400.
	TOTAL DENTAL EXPENSES	$18,900.

What did this bill of $18,900 *actually* cost Bryce Robertson? Let's subtract the amount covered by his dental insurance.

Insurance coverage for Bryce Robertson	$1,000.
Insurance coverage for Mary Robertson	1,000.
Insurance coverage for Bryce Jr.	500.
Insurance coverage for Jean	500.
TOTAL INSURANCE COVERAGE	$3,000.

Therefore, the amount due to be paid by Bryce Robertson turned out to be $15,900. In his tax bracket, this resulted in *a tax saving of approximately $8,000,* leaving an actual outlay of $7,900.*

---

*This is a hypothetical case and all figures are approximate.

That's dentistry for the rich and the super rich! What do the poor and the unaware get?

Dentistry For The Poor and Unaware

Contrast the dental care of the rich Bryce Robertson family of Short Hills, New Jersey, with the poor William Jackson* family, who live a scant ten miles away in the "Down Neck" section of Newark. Unlike the five acre estate of the Robertsons, the Jacksons occupy five rooms of a six family frame tenement. Instead of manicured lawns and a swimming pool, the approach to the Jackson's apartment is garbage cans, noisy neighbors, and a view of the city's teeming streets. For the past ten years, Bill Jackson has been trying to move his family to a better neighborhood. But with the recession, inflation, and some bad breaks, he hasn't been able to swing it.

Bill Jackson, 42, works for a local construction firm as a mason's helper. He earns about $250 a week when he works, but he doesn't always get a full week's work. His yearly gross income is just under $10,000. Since he's not in a union, he doesn't have any health insurance — no medical, hospital, or dental benefits. The only time Bill was in a country club was when he redid the brick patio off the main dining room of The Penbrook Golf Club. His recreation consists of beers and a night out bowling "with the boys." His beat up Chevy has over 65,000 miles on it, but he figures it's good for another couple of years. His limited education and skills have Bill pretty well "locked in" to his current social and economic level.

His wife Anita, 38, is a part-time cashier at the local supermarket. Because she's only part-time, Anita is not entitled to any fringe benefits or insurance coverage. Her annual salary is about $2500. Over the years, Anita has tried to "help out" the family income with a series of part-time factory jobs. She has always been on an hourly basis, and never earned more than $4,000 in any given year. She shops for her clothes at Korvettes, and takes the bus to work. Her Thursday night Bingo Game is her major recreation.

Like the Robertson family, the Jacksons also have two children. Jimmy, 18, is a high school senior who pumps gas at a nearby Getty

*All names are fictitious.

station after school. Jimmy's grades have never been good, so he enrolled in "the work-study program" that allows him to leave school every day at noon to go to work. He gets high school credits for his time spent on the job, and he is able to pay for his own needs with the money he earns. Recently, he bought a motorcycle that seems to eat up all his spare cash.

May, 16, is a high school sophomore and is also in "the work-study program," working as a stock clerk in a Newark department store. She has emotional problems and hates school.

Dental History of The Jacksons

(Bill) Bill Jackson had been going to the same dentist whenever he had a toothache. With each toothache he usually lost a tooth. Most of his back teeth are missing. Some front teeth have holes in them. A lot of his co-workers and friends are pretty much in the same position. Bill plans to have all his teeth out when more of them are lost. Then, he believes, his dental problems will be over. He heard of a place in Pennsylvania where he can get a full set of dentures cheap ($150). One of his bowling buddies went there and told him about it.

(Anita) Anita Jackson claims she comes from a family of "bad teeth." Although she's only 38, she wears a full upper denture and a large lower partial denture. Ten years ago, she went to a dentist who put her to sleep. She woke up with all her upper teeth removed. She's proud of the fact that she was "lucky enough" to save some bottom teeth for hooks. She heard that full lower dentures were very hard to wear. Most of her dental knowledge comes from co-workers, friends, and relatives. Both her older sisters already wear full plates and have advised her, "We got bad teeth. Don't spend no money on 'em."

(Jimmy) Jimmy first visited the dentist when he was eight years old. He had a terrible toothache and a swollen jaw. His father had to hold him down while the dentist extracted his permanent six year molar. Bill Jackson thought it was only a baby tooth. The entire episode was a bad experience, and to this day Jimmy trembles with fear at the thought of going to a dentist.

Now 18, Jimmy is already missing five permanent teeth. He had been going to the city dental clinic for a while, but hated the long waits on the hard benches in the waiting room. Each time he went to the city clinic, he got a different dentist who usually bawled him out for not brushing his teeth. Jimmy hasn't been to the dentist in the last two years. He eats plenty of candy and drinks lots of soda pop. He brushes his teeth occasionally, and he's pretty sure that one day he'll "get 'em all out." If he had to choose between spending money to save a tooth or buying a new shield for his motorcycle, the shield would win hands down.

(May) May, age 16, was told by the school dentist three years ago that she needed orthodontic treatments. At that time, her mother took May to a dental school clinic, where she was advised that the waiting period was two years for orthodontic patients. May never had the work done. Consequently, her upper front teeth have become very "buck." Because of this marked protrusion of her upper front teeth, May cannot get her lips together to make a normal lip seal. This condition has caused her to become a habitual mouth breather, which resulted in frequent upper respiratory infections. Furthermore, the kids have nicknamed her "Bugs Bunny." This dental-facial defect has caused her much emotional trauma. She has become shy and introverted. When she does smile (which is rare), her hand is always near her mouth, a habit she developed to hide her teeth. She never speaks up in class, and her attendance and grades have suffered because of this problem. Her young life is on a downward spiral.

• • • • •

For the Bill Jackson family, dental care revolves around neglect, toothaches, and extractions. Their dental health care is a hundred light years away from the Robertson family.

Most of us are neither as rich as the Robertsons nor as poor as the Jacksons. Money helps — there's no denying that. But so does being an informed consumer who can make intelligent choices. No matter what your income is, $10,000 or $100,000, you can learn *how to save your teeth and your money.*

11
The Newest in Dentistry:
Dentistry of the Future

Dentistry of the past has been anchored to a mechanical concept of filling teeth, extractions, and making plates. As recently as 20 years ago, parents assumed it was a waste of money to take care of their children's baby teeth. Today, however, the old fashioned dental office located over a pharmacy is rapidly vanishing. Like the model T Ford, the drab one chair office is no longer being built.

What's in the future for dentistry? What are the issues and trends that will affect your teeth and your pocketbook?

Private Group Practices

The young dentist starting out today is better informed, better educated, and has higher expectations than the generation that graduated before him. Many of the new graduates are choosing to work themselves into *group practices* of several established dentists, instead of starting out with that old, one chair office over the pharmacy. There are considerable advantages for the young dentist, but *there are also advantages for you.* Groups of dentists, often specialists in different aspects of dentistry, can give you a more comprehensive quality treatment, and with several other colleagues looking over their shoulders, the quality of their work is likely to be high. Groups can afford better diagnostic tools, more up-to-date equipment, and more efficient care, so you're likely to get a better value for your dollar, too, although the actual cost of your dentistry may not be less.

National Health Insurance

Some people believe that private group dental practices can't handle tomorrow's needs. They feel a comprehensive dental care package, *with Uncle Sam as the group,* is the only answer. Such a system would use clinics administered by a National Health Program, and it would be available to everyone, not just the poor or the elderly, and perhaps be open weekends and evenings. Private dental practices would still exist, but a national health care system which included dental care would cover everyone. Who would pay the bill? You would, of course, through additional taxes.

Organized dentistry is *against* such a system. The American Dental Association, individual dentists, and some non-professionals feel it will result in bureaucratic, low quality, red tape dentistry. As evidence, they point to the low quality of dentistry in other countries where a national health program is run — England, for example. And they point with pride to the high quality, superior dentistry under our system of private practice. They feel their fears are well founded in the overwhelming reports of Medicare abuses, Welfare cheating, administrative waste, and disreputable government practices that cost American taxpayers billions a year when the government takes over.

Those who are *for* it think the private dental group practices are only a placebo. Many groups, they say, are actually conglomerates out for their own good. They are in business together to reap greater profits, take time off, and increase their productivity. They feel group practices are not the answer, are too costly, and do not reach enough people (especially the poor).

The question of National Health Insurance is tangled in a mass of charges and countercharges, fears, and accusations. It's a political hot potato. Certainly, many of these fears are grounded in solid experience with government intervention. On the other hand, the present system of private practice, whether by an individual dentist or a group, is *not* delivering dental care to enough people at a cost we can afford. Right now, even with President Carter in the White House, it certainly doesn't look as if National Health Insurance is about to be hatched.

Private Insurance Plans

The tidal wave of dental insurance plans is awakening a new interest in dental care and reaching out to include a vast number of people who formerly neglected their teeth. As recently as 1965, less than 2 million Americans had any kind of insurance for dental work. Today, about 30 million are already included, and by 1980, the American Dental Association estimates the total will rise to about 60 million.

That means *more dental work for more people.* The extension of dental insurance coverage to millions of workers through their unions and employers has caused the dentist many problems. The profession complains loudly about the burden of the paper-work, the intervention of unqualified insurance adjusters who approve or disapprove claims, and the slow moving bureaucracy administering the plans.

Still, most dentists agree that prepaid dental insurance represents a milestone for everyone involved, and that it will be good for both dentist and patient. Unions and employers also give it a positive vote. The cost to them runs slightly over $10 a month for an employee and his dependents, and is a tremendous fringe benefit to offer any employee or union member. It looks like *dental insurance is one of the newest trends in dentistry, and is here to stay.*

Credit

Millions of dental consumers are now demanding better and more comprehensive treatment. How will they pay for it? Credit! Credit has become a way of life in America. Car rentals, vacations, hotels, restaurants, and clothing can be taken care of on credit. Why not dental bills?

Everyone is familiar with Master Charge, American Express, and Diners Club. Every day consumers flash their credit cards to charge gasoline at the pumps, to make a phone call, or to buy a book or a broiler. Credit has become an essential part of our lifestyle, and it's the rare person who pays cash for everything he buys.

In the future, the American consumer may soon extend his credit cards to pay his physician and his dentist. Already, a number of state medical associations have endorsed accepting approved bank cards from patients. And why not? Physicians and dentists, like other businesspeople, are in competition for your credit dollar. They provide a service, but they also have to collect the funds. In the future, when you receive your dental bill, you may be able to snap back, "Charge it, please!" and flash your card.

Ever notice how charge customers get better treatment in department stores? Ever wonder why you have more clout when you charge something for credit or when you register a complaint if you're a charge customer? The same may be true for dental consumers. The patient who charges may also receive better treatment, and his complaint may register just a bit louder if his bills are charged.

The Public Policy Dentist

Most of us think of the dentist as the person in the white jacket who fills our teeth. However, a new breed of dentist is emerging today: The Public Policy Dentist. These men and women do *not* work on individual patients, as your own dentist does. Instead, they concern themselves with the many broad issues involving *patient's rights.*

The public policy dentist will be the guiding force in finding and implementing ways to give you better dentistry at lower costs. He will investigate quality dental care for the poor, evaluate dental materials and devices for safety, implement peer review, and lobby for the redistribution of dentists to areas of greater need. This corps of men and women will make political and social decisions that will directly affect the quality of the dental work you receive, and the money you're going to spend to get it.

Here are some of those broad issues you and the public policy dentist will be concerned with, because they affect your dental health and your pocketbook.

State Board Licensing

In order for your dentist to practice, he must be licensed by the State. The fact that he has spent four years in dental school, undergoing intensive study and constant examination, does *not* permit him to hang out his shingle and go to work. Only the approval of the State Board can license the dental school graduate to practice.

Everyone talks about the State Boards. Critics loudly proclaim them unfair, unnecessary, discriminatory, outdated, and even useless in measuring dental competence. But the attempts to banish them appear doomed at this moment. What does that mean to you?

In 1880, when State Boards were born, there was a good reason for them — to protect the public from dentists trained in unsupervised schools. But with accreditation of dental schools by the American Dental Association and the written national examinations, the whole business of state licensing has become a hotly debated subject.

Many contend State Boards simply protect the economic interest of dentists. *They check competition, not competency,* by restricting the number of dentists practicing in their state. The less dentists around, the higher the fees you have to pay. That follows the basic law of supply and demand.

In 1972, an American Dental Association Poll showed 70% of its members favored reciprocity — meaning a dentist in one state could practice in another *without State Board Exams.* Nationwide reciprocity based on national standards could help relieve the shortage of dentists in tightly controlled states. For example, Mississippi does *not* accept other state licenses, and has only 1 dentist for every 3900 people. Connecticut, a state which *does* accept some other state licenses, has 1 dentist for every 1500 people.

Already, 21 states and the District of Columbia have some limited reciprocity in effect. This could mean lowering the costs of your dental care.

Recently, the Consumers Union filed a suit challenging Pennsylvania's exclusion of lay persons (that means you, the consumer) from State Boards for optometrists. It was the first suit on behalf of consumers. Another thrust for consumers came in Princeton, when New Jersey dentists met with consumer advocates to discuss the inclusion of lay persons on their State Board.

Many people feel dentists are looking out for dentists when they regulate policies on their State Boards, and that consumers should be included on those State Boards *to look out for their consumer interests.* The whole question of State Boards is bound to be resolved in the future. As a dental consumer, you'll want to understand this issue and look out for your own interests.

Redistribution of Dentists

The problem of maldistribution of dentists and physicians appears to be a very real problem in our country today. In 1973, California had 265 physicians for every 100,000 population, while South Dakota had only 87 physicians for the same 100,000 population. This disparity is even greater than the figures indicate, because doctors tend to locate in urban areas at the expense of rural sections. What can be done about it?

> **One Billion Cavities**
>
> *It has been estimated that if every dentist spent 24 hours a day, every day, for one year, just filling cavities, there would still be one billion cavities left unfilled in the United States alone.*

Some people advocate that doctors should be drafted to serve areas where there is a medical-dental shortage, in return for the government financing their education. That means a medical or dental student educated at government expense can either repay the cost of his education, or serve for several years in a designated area.

Senator Edward M. Kennedy believes every American has the right to health care, and he proposed a *universal draft for all medical school graduates*. But opponents ask whether doctors serving against their will can give adequate service. Should they be singled out to relieve maldistribution in their professions when lawyers, pharmacists, and engineers are not?

The American Student Dental Association claims manpower shortages do *not* exist, and oversupply will be a problem in the 1980s. Yet pockets of poor, rural areas are virtually without health care.

Others feel we must *increase the number of dental schools* which turn away thousands of applicants every year. They say we must turn out more dentists. Many students, harassed by dental school faculties, complain bitterly about the amount of trivia and useless information jammed into their curriculum. They believe curriculum revision and judicious pruning would turn out better dentists in shorter time and make way for more dentists to graduate.

In the meantime, in an effort to bring dental services where the need is greatest, *mobile trailers* are being tried in remote areas. In Utah, for example, at Navajo Mountain and Montezuma Creek, two sub-satellite clinics were set up by Loma Linda dental students. In the Hartford, Connecticut area, "Smilemobile," a 29 foot van which cost over $30,000, visited 9,000 schoolchildren.

In 1972, the mean net average for a private dentist in the United States was $35,698. We can expect that figure to be even higher today. Obviously dentists come out pretty well on the economic ladder. Whether patients in rural and poverty areas come out decently is another question. If you live in a rural or isolated area, you may be getting short changed.

Peer Review

How do you know if you're getting what you paid for? You're not a dentist, so you don't have the professional expertise to make critical judgments. Even if you do suspect you were short changed, barring a flagrant abuse or obvious rip-off, it's hard to pin it down. Lay persons, it seems, can never be absolutely sure the quality of their dentistry is satisfactory.

Is there any other way by which dentists' competency is checked? Or can any dentist — even your own — get away with disreputable work with impunity? That's where peer review comes in. *It means dentists checking on other dentists,* weeding out the incompetents, reporting the frauds, and criticizing their own colleagues. It may be possible, but it's not easy. Why? Because most doctors are reluctant to report the incompetent work they see, and this, perhaps, is the greatest obstacle to better regulation of the profession.

A recent case that received great notoriety was "the curare case," in which a New Jersey physician practicing in a well known hospital allegedly murdered hospital patients with curare injections. He continued to practice for ten years before his license was suspended. This veil of silence can shield the incompetent, the alcoholic, even the murderer.

Are dental licenses ever revoked? *The New York Times* reported that out of the 320,000 physicians practicing in the United States in the years 1971-1974, on the average, only 72 medical licenses were revoked. In attempting to establish similar records for dentists, we wrote to the American Dental Association asking for the number of dental licenses revoked in past years. Our first letter received the following reply:

To our knowledge, revocations by state boards of dentistry during the past few years have not been compiled.

Unwilling to accept that cursory reply, we wrote another letter asking the question again. This time we were more insistent. We said:

Please send ANY available information that your office might have that deals with methods of policing or disciplining dentists for incompetence or dishonesty on national and state levels. It is hard to believe that NO information exists on the number of dentists who have had their licenses revoked.

The second reply from the American Dental Association was merely a hand written note, jotted off at the bottom of our own letter, repeating the first reply. It said:

To my* knowledge, the information you are seeking has not been compiled.

We did receive, at our request, a list of individual state offices, so we could track it down state by state. The list was titled "State and Regional Dental Agency Secretaries." Since we could get no answer from the American Dental Association, we wrote 51 separate letters to each state and the District of Columbia. We have received the following replies.

Dental Licenses Revoked

ARIZONA	In the last 5 years, 3 licenses were revoked, *all* for commission of a felony.
CALIFORNIA	In 1974, there were 6 suspensions, 1 revocation, and 13 probations.
CONNECTICUT	No information given.

* Letter signed B.J. Crawford.

NEW JERSEY	In 1975, of the 14 matters considered, 2 licenses were revoked: 1 for drug abuse; the other for improper work. In 1973-74, 1 license was revoked for sexual assault. Other matters were dismissed or financial restitution was imposed.
NEW YORK	From 1971-1976, there were 4 licenses revoked for charges such as immoral conduct, conviction of a crime, fraud and deceit, and unprofessional conduct.
MICHIGAN	In the past 4 years, there were 3 "suspensions:" 1 for fraud; 1 for a felony; and 1 for unprofessional conduct. There were also 5 revocations: 1 for a sex offense; 1 for incompetency; and 3 for drug addiction.
MISSOURI	No information available.
OKLAHOMA	From 1972 to the present, there were 8 "suspensions:" 2 for criminal convictions; 1 for evading income tax; 1 for false insurance claims; 2 for unauthorized acts by auxiliaries; 2 for drug addiction. Only 1 of the 8 "suspensions" was a permanent revocation.
SOUTH DAKOTA	No licenses revoked.
TEXAS	From 1972-76, there were 13 licenses revoked and 21 suspended for periods of 1-10 years. The offenses ranged from illegal signs to hefty crimes like burglary, kidnapping, and sexual abuse of a child.
UTAH	No revocations; 1 suspension.
WEST VIRGINIA	"Information is confidential"
WYOMING	No licenses revoked.

To summarize, of the 51 letters we sent out, only 13 states replied. Of those, 3 states (Connecticut, Missouri, and West Virginia) gave no information; and 3 states (South Dakota, Utah and Wyoming) claimed they had no revocations. Therefore, only 7 states answered that they *had* revoked some dental licenses: Arizona, California, New Jersey, New York, Michigan, Oklahoma, and Texas.

It is interesting to note that when dental licenses were revoked, they were often for major crimes like drug addiction, fraud, burglary, kidnapping, and sex offenses. No license was specifically revoked for a simple consumer concern like overcharging or performing plain bad work!

In other words, if your dentist is a rapist, drug addict, or kidnapper, his license could be taken away. But if he pulls the wrong tooth or bills you for work he never did, he may go on practicing for years undetected and free of censure. That could be costing you plenty!

Not All Doctors Are Honest

Senator Frank E. Moss, Chairman of the Senate subcommittee on Long Term Care, has charged that more than $300 million dollars a year in Medicare fraud can be attributed to doctors.

Continuing Education

Once a dentist has a license to practice, even if that license is 50 years old, *he has no re-examinations to take forever after.* In other words, a dentist who received his license half a century ago is still licensed to practice, in spite of the fact that he might be light years away from the exploding scientific strides of today.

If you have any doubts about your own dentist, don't be afraid to ask when he graduated, and if he's taken any courses since then. The up-to-date professional will be proud to tell about his additional studies, and you're likely to notice it in the superior work you get.

Some states do make feeble efforts to have their dentists keep up with the times through additional education. But for the most part, the requirements are meager and voluntary.

In reply to our request for information on continuing education for dentists, the American Dental Association sent us this list (dated October, 1973) of states which require continuing education for dental relicensure. The list was headed by this statement:

"The following information is not completely definitive since this office has on occasion, in the course of compiling this data,

received conflicting statements from sources that are equally authoritative."

>Kansas — 30 hours every 3 years
>Kentucky — 20 points every 2 years
>Minnesota — 40 hours every 5 years
>North Dakota — 20 hours every 5 years
>South Dakota — 20 hours every 5 years

We do not know if any dentist has lost his license for failure to comply!

Dental Auxiliary

In the past, a dentist who practiced solo in his own one chair office performed like a one-man band. He answered the phone, took and developed your X rays, cleaned your teeth, sent out bills, collected money, made appointments, and performed every single function of running an office without the help of a single auxiliary person.

Today, it is the rare dental office that doesn't employ some auxiliary personnel to work alongside the dentist. Sometimes in large group practices, the number of auxiliaries can exceed the number of dentists. There may be, for example, in a group of four dentists: two dental hygienists to clean teeth and explain prevention and home care; a dental receptionist to make appointments and keep records; a business manager to order supplies and coordinate all aspects of the practice; and four chairside dental assistants (one for each dentist), making a total of eight auxiliary personnel.

What does that mean to you, the quality of the dentistry you will get, and the costs you will pay? In most cases, it means more efficiency, which could be passed on to you as savings. Specially trained oral hygienists, for example, will clean your teeth, in many cases with results superior to a dentist's. These oral hygienists have even proved capable of producing high quality fillings. Where? In New Zealand, where the dental nurse concept has proven effective in reducing the number of unfilled teeth in school children. Why not use this concept in the United States? It could cut costs for you and your family.

Future dentistry could incorporate the "dental nurse" as a powerful adjunct to ease dental shortages in such critical areas as inner cities and isolated rural pockets of poverty. Studies of dental nurses trained in the New Zealand method at the Forsyth Dental Center in Boston show that after only 26 weeks, they could perform as competently as recent graduate dentists in certain areas.

It seems so simple, and yet the expanding role of the dental auxiliary is viewed with suspicion by many dentists. Why let these auxiliaries take over their turf. Once an auxiliary is allowed to take an X ray, give an injection, or fill a baby tooth, dentists feel their professional position is threatened. There are also some fears for their economic security.

In spite of this, *the concept of team dentistry* (the dentist and his assistants working together) can make dental care more available and less costly to you. If more dental nurses are trained, more work can be done. And if that training produces good work in a short time, your dental costs could come down. Isn't that what every consumer is looking for?

The dental nurse concept has spread to Malaysia, Indonesia, Ceylon, England, Columbia, Cuba, Jamaica, Ghana, Hong Kong, Korea, Laos, Senegal, South Viet Nam, Thailand, Uganda, and most recently, Canada. But within the United States, the dental nurse is still not a legal concept, except as a teaching experience.

We accept a physician who routinely delegates work to competent medical auxiliary. Why not accept dental auxiliary to assume similar technical procedures? This can only elevate the dentist to diagnostician and specialist. And it can mean more efficient, less costly dental care for you.

Women in Dentistry

Throughout this book we have consistently referred to the dentist as "he." In no way was this meant to discount or depreciate the value of women in dentistry. We have used the "he" for two reasons: first, because the alternative "he or she" and "his or hers" makes clumsy, wordy reading; and second, because the obvious and regrettable fact is that women in the United States have been excluded, by and large, from the dental profession. It was only those rare women with exceptional scholarship and burning ambition who made it through dental school to hang out their shingle. Even today, with the feminist movement making great strides to correct inequalities of the past, dental schools accept only a handful of women, and women dentists are rare birds.

Although the Health Manpower (*MAN*power?) Development Training Act of 1971 requires professional schools to provide equal opportunities for women, it is glaringly apparent that this still has not been implemented in the dental profession. Obviously, young women of considerable talents are willing to accept the challenges of a career in dentistry. Yet it is disturbing that dentistry as a career is still not really open to women. Why?

We cannot, in fairness, lay all the blame on dental schools, though they certainly come in for their share of the blame. A significant factor is that girls at a very early age are steered into traditionally female roles in the health sciences: nurse, dental assistant, medical secretary. As a result, *only 2% of dentists in our country are women.*

In European countries, women contribute a significantly larger proportion to the dental population. Half the dentists in Greece are women; and in Poland, the USSR, and Finland, about 80% are women. In Caracas, Venezuela, 90% of the city's dentists are women.

The truth is that many women possess qualities that can only enhance their effectiveness as dentists: deep warmth, compassion, and sympathy for the sick and troubled; plus a clearer understanding of how to deal with children.

Dr. Eva Kornblith, the first woman periodontist in New Jersey, must have been a pioneer when she entered dental school, over 60 years ago, in 1916. Still vital at 84, Dr. Kornblith recalled how she combined a career and a happy family life, long before the heyday of the liberated woman.

"If I had to advise a young woman who was interested in dentistry today," she said, "I would recommend it very highly."

After 52 years of practice in Newark, New Jersey, this pioneer woman is a model and inspiration for any young woman considering dentistry today. She speaks eloquently for *woman power in dentistry!*

Advertising

If dentists were to advertise, would that affect your pocketbook? Would fees come down? Would it help you to know which dentists charge what fees, and which are specialists? Or would it lead to cut-throat Madison Avenue techniques, TV jingles, and fourth class ads squashed into your mailbox?

In Alaska, a proposal was drafted "to eliminate restraints traditionally placed on members of certain professions so that consumers may have access to information concerning services and related fees." What's it all about?

Recent, new interpretations of price fixing under the Sherman Antitrust Act led the Federal Trade Commission (FTC) to file a complaint against the American Medical Association. Both the American Medical Association and the American Dental Association have consistently banned advertising by their members. The FTC contends that this restricts competition, and that as a result, consumers (that means you) are deprived of information to help them select a doctor.

Should the ban against advertising be lifted (and it seems unlikely, given the strong opposition of the American Dental Association) it's doubtful that a whole slew of dentists will rush forth to go that route. Many doctors, like Raymond T. Holden, Chairman of the American Medical Association's Board of Trustees, feel that "advertising by a professional is the very antithesis of professionalism. Physicians should not solicit patients." Dentists apparently feel the same way. To the question "Do you favor advertising by the learned professions?", 92% said NO.

The FTC feels differently. They think advertising probably would have a great impact on the fees you're paying. Their philosophy is that disclosure, as through advertising, is healthy and beneficial to the public. Will flashing neon signs blaze from professional buildings across the country? We doubt it.

Can Dentists Advertise?

Dentist Joan C. Staker has decided to put it to the test in the Federal District Court. Dr. Staker charges that state rules deny her the right to advertise her specialty of orthodontics in the Yellow Pages, and this violates her constitutional rights. The Long Island, New York dentist is asking a cool million in damages.

However, the Supreme Court has already ruled that professional pharmacists may advertise the prices of prescription drugs, a ruling that may save consumers tens of millions of dollars a year. The American Medical Association ban against doctors advertising is still unyielding, but it is softening. They now allow their members to advertise their names, the types of practices, location of their offices, hours available, and "other useful information that will enable the public to make a more informed choice of physician."

Before the forces of consumerism emerged, advertising was considered taboo in "the learned professions." But right now, lawyers are leaning toward it, too. If that happens, who knows? Next to tout his services could be your dentist!

> **Dentist Advertises on TV**
>
> Dr. Don Norwood, an Indianapolis dentist, thinks dentists "have a monopoly worse than the oil companies." So he's gone on TV to hawk his orthodontic fees. His $2000 a month radio and TV ads have paid off. He sees as many as 60 patients some days.

Group practices, National Health Insurance, private insurance, the Public Policy Dentist, State Boards, credit, peer review, redistribution of dentists, continuing education, dental auxiliary, women in dentistry, advertising . . . what does any of that have to do with you? Aren't those political issues a long distance from your wallet and your teeth? What possible difference can they make to you, the dental consumer?

We think *they make a great deal of difference.* They color your world, because they affect the kind of dental care you're likely to get and the bill that follows it up. If you are aware of these issues, you can affect legislation, lobby for your own interests, press for your own patient bill of rights. You won't be a sitting duck, buying a blind item, unable to understand what you're paying for and afraid to speak out.

Why leave your dental destiny in the hands of others? Take charge of your life and demand what is rightfully yours — *a fair shake as a dental consumer.*

So much for the political issues that affect you. What about the *scientific advancements* that are about to be hatched? What can you hope for in the future? What's on the horizon that will make your visits to the dentist more pleasant, more beneficial, and more economical?

X rays

Better and more sophisticated X rays that are faster and safer are already in use. Many dentists are also using the *new Panorex-type X ray,* which gives them additional specific information for their diagnosis. Today, progressive dentists can take a panoramic shot of the entire jawbone area, including the sinuses. This picture enables them to measure exactly the location of existing teeth, and also *to predict where other teeth will erupt.*

The panagram also helps the dentist determine whether or not there is room enough for the mouth to accommodate the new teeth into the jawbone. The orthodontist whose panagram indicates dim prospects for a well positioned set of teeth, may decide to extract selected permanent teeth to make room for the erupting ones.

So these new advanced X rays remove the guesswork and speculation, and make your dentist's diagnosis and treatment more accurate.

Clear Plastic Brackets

Another advance in orthodontics is the new fixed appliances. *Plastic orthodontic attachments that are almost invisible* have replaced the old silver "Brace Face" look. These nearly invisible appliances are bonded directly to the surface of each tooth, eliminating the need for unsightly, heavy metal bands.

The improved appliances are more comfortable to wear because they take up less room in your mouth and feel less bulky. And since they're easier for the dentist to apply, they mean you'll spend less time in the dental chair. This could be reflected in an overall lower cost to you.

Computer Forecasting

If you think computers are used only to tally your department store bills, you're mistaken. A computer may soon tell dentists whether or not a child should have his budding wisdom tooth extracted to avoid the further complications of impaction at a later date.

A dental researcher at U.C.L.A., Patrick Turley, has come up with *a forecasting system*. How does it work? Data, taken from a child's X ray when he is 8 or 9, is added to some simple measurements of his jaw and fed into the computer. The machine, primed with the research, then advises the dentist whether or not the child is likely to run into trouble when he hits college age. If the computer's outlook is negative, the third molar bud can be removed — a simple procedure that could avoid more complicated surgery once the wisdom tooth is fully grown and becomes impacted. It could save you money to have it done at 9 instead of 19.

Sonar Devices

Not only are computer principles being used in dentistry, but so are sonar principles. New sonar-like devices now employ sound waves to measure distances in the mouth. They can now *determine, electronically, the depth of a periodontal pocket or the length of a root canal.*

They utilize the very same principles that a submarine uses to scan the oceans for the presence and location of another ship. Just as the computer helped take the guesswork out of diagnosis of tooth eruption, so these sonar devices take the guesswork out of diagnosis for the periodontist and the endodontist.

These devices are bound to save the dentist time and increase his accuracy. This could mean better dental care for you.

Fiber Optic Lights

There is now a new, advanced method of lighting your mouth. Tiny strands of glass fibers can now conduct light directly into your mouth for better visibility. This is the method called fiber optic lighting, where the main light source comes from a remote location, and is then transmitted through *flexible glass strands* gathered into bundles. Small enough to even enter a tooth socket, they can help the dentist locate a tiny broken root tip. They can even be beamed *directly* into the nerve canal to increase visibility when the endodontist is working there.

The major feature of this type of light is that *no heat or electricity is given off* at the tip of the strand located in your mouth. Therefore, there is no discomfort or danger.

Fiber optic lighting is also small enough to be placed on the high speed drill, acting as a "headlight," with the beam focused on the tip of the drill. This brings an intense light to bear directly on the area your dentist is working on.

Tooth Banks

Swedish researchers have successfully developed a *technique for freezing an extracted tooth, for a year or more,* for implantation later on. Using this new technique, it is possible to extract a poorly positioned tooth, along with its root tissue, and reinsert it at a different site on the same person — or perhaps even into another person's mouth.

Dr. P. Otteskog, of the Karolina Institute of Stockholm, uses a liquid nitrogen device to freeze the tooth and drop temperatures down to minus 280 degrees. This dental deep freeze could lead to the establishment of tooth banks.

You've heard of eyebanks and sperm banks. Soon we may have tooth banks, where donar and recipient would be carefully matched. In need of a second molar? Phone the tooth bank.

Saliva Tests

Researchers at Columbia University have devised a test you can't flunk. Dr. David Abelson and Dr. Michael Marder have found that changes in your saliva could provide important tip-offs to doctors. These saliva tests may give diagnostic *clues to a wide variety of physical disorders,* from cirrhosis of the liver to diabetes and hypertension. Dentists are already using the sphygmomanometer (blood pressure cuff) in their offices to screen high blood pressure in dental patients. The saliva test could provide additional data. For example, their studies show that diabetics have an abnormal amount of calcium in their saliva.

The composition of saliva may also reflect different hormonal states, like pregnancy or menopause. Like the familiar blood test, the saliva test could become another routine test for diagnosis.

Tooth Implants

It has been said: "It is not enough to add years to life, but rather life to years."

Today, people are enjoying longevity far beyond that of previous generations. Some of these senior citizens may be physically fit for their advanced years, but many suffer from unsatisfactory, conventional dentures. Here is where tooth implants may come in to make a contribution.

Implants are not for everybody, but *may be indicated in a denture patient who simply cannot adjust to wearing a denture.* What are the alternatives for these unhappy patients?

1. Not wear their denture at all — go toothless.
2. Suffer with uncomfortable dentures they wear only when they "go out."
3. Seek a dentist who feels a dental implant can be successful for them.

What is a dental implant? Dental implantology is a method of imbedding metallic or other biocompatible materials directly into the jawbone, onto which artificial teeth are fastened. That means the *implants are not removable, but fixed; and the artificial teeth built over them feel and function like natural teeth.* A simple implant could take only 30 minutes and be done with a local anesthetic. Cost? Not much more than normal bridgework.

The good news about dental implants is that they will not decay like natural teeth. However, bone resorption (shrinkage), similar to periodontal disease, can still occur and cause the implants to loosen.

Actually, implants have been done since 1949, and many are now in the mouth over 25 years. Today they are becoming more and more common. About 13,000 dentists have already taken courses in implantology. Much success has been reported, and implant techniques have been refined through research in implant material (vitalium, carbon vitreous materials, and hydrothermally treated coral).

Not every dentist is trained and equipped to do dental implants. And they don't work for everybody. But the person who can smile, laugh, talk, eat, kiss, and be comfortable with this type of replacement becomes a missionary for implantology. The acceptance of oral implantology is becoming more and more widespread, and it promises to play a larger role in future dentistry.

Dental Vaccines

Today's decay control methods such as fluorides, pit and fissure sealants, and plaque control are only "holding devices." What's coming up in the future? Perhaps the total elimination of decay by means of *a simple "shot" — a vaccination against the acid producing bacteria that settle in dental plaque and attack the enamel of your teeth.*

Researchers in the United States and other countries are already at work on this project, and the results are encouraging. Professor Thomas Lehner of Guy's Hospital in London reports a decrease in cavities in animals injected with a heat killed strain of *Streptococcus mutans,* the prime decay causing microorganism in human mouths. And Dr. Fred G. Emmings in New York reports that injections into salivary glands of animals stimulates the production of antibodies in the saliva. At the National Institute of Dental Research in Bethesda, Maryland, where researchers are working to immunize rats against *Streptococcus mutans,* tests showed that the immunized rats developed high levels of antibodies in their blood and saliva.

Any research on humans? A British oral surgeon, Dr. Geoffrey E. Smith, claims his 12 years of research have turned up a vaccine that will cut decay in children up to 90%.

Right now dental decay is not a killing or even crippling disease. But it is responsible for considerable pain and costly repairs to 95% of the population. Perhaps if all these research projects on animals come to fruition, and can be successfully applied to humans of all ages, decay may all but disappear. If this comes to pass, dental cavities, like polio and smallpox, will be relegated to the pages of history books. In the future, a simple "shot" could save your teeth and your money.

Forensic Dentistry

Ever wonder how they identify the bodies in cases of disasters or catastrophes? For victims of such disasters, *the dentist is the key figure in identification.*

The increase in international air and sea travel within the last 20 years may be responsible for the progress of forensic dentistry (*the positive identification of a person through dental records*). All people exhibit individualities in their bite, but the dentist is the one professional to distinguish between similar bites. Bodies mutilated beyond recognition, even down to fingerprints, may be identified through their dental records.

Even in cases not involving air crashes or natural catastrophes, the forensic dentist may be called upon to testify. For example, he may testify in a murder trial to clearly identify the murderer. In Scotland, to cite a specific case, the accused was found guilty mainly on the evidence of a London dentist, Dr. Warren Harvey, who had been given photographs of bite marks on the victim's body. Of 29 plaster dental models given him, Dr. Harvey identified only one set — the accused murderer — through distinctive characteristics of the right upper and lower canines.

In November, 1965, near the Greater Cincinnati Airport, a Boeing 727 crashed, killing 58 of the 62 people aboard. The victims were identified through the efforts of forensic dentistry.

In most cases of catastrophe, identification via fingerprints is of little use. Here's where the forensic dentist steps in. Through his investigation, identification by means of dental records can usually tip the scale of the investigation and clearly establish the victim's identity.

> **Two Families Claim Same Body in Air Crash**
>
> *In April, 1968, a South African Airways 707 crashed, killing 122 people. In one instance, the body of a young woman was claimed by two families. It took a dental chart to make the correct identification.*

Acupuncture Anesthesia

Until recently, acupuncture was practically unheard of in the United States. To most people it seemed a kind of Chinese folk medicine, and it was largely unknown or misunderstood in America. Many equated it with charlatanism, voodoo, and the old rip-off.

How it works is still a mystery to American physicians and dentists, and for that matter, Chinese doctors can't explain it either.* It has to do with what the Chinese call *yin* and *yang* — the positive and negative forces — and the acupuncturist, not necessarily a doctor, manipulates needles at points on or near "meridians" of the body to restore the balance between the *yin* and *yang*. The needle may be twirled by hand or, in some cases, electrical impulses are added to the needles. In fact, recently acupuncturists have used electrodes without needles to impart electrical impulses directly to the skin.

Does acupuncture work for the suppression of pain? It is already being used to relieve the pain of arthritis, bursitis, temporomandibular joint pain, headaches, and neuralgias. It has also been used in anesthetizing patients in certain types of operations, notably head, throat and chest surgery. But others still feel it's inferior to the local anesthetics presently used for dental operations.

Those who tout it feel it might be useful to avoid allergic reactions and side effects of traditional analgesics; that it has some application for patients in poor health where general anesthesia is a greater risk; or for those who fear local anesthesia via injection.

Is it for you? If you think you're a candidate for acupuncture anesthesia, talk to your dentist and see how he feels about it. There aren't many dentists around who practice it, but if you're absolutely set on the idea, you may be able to make a connection through a dental school or teaching hospital.

Hypnodontics

Hypnotism generally conjures up the image of parlor games, the occult, and surrender of the will. For most people, it is suspect, and they scoff at it with the same mild amusement given fortune tellers and tea leaf readers. Recently, however, it has gained some limited acceptance for applications in medicine, psychiatry, psychoanalysis, and dentistry.

In dentistry, *hypnotism can be used for pain control — thus the word hypnodontics*. Like acupuncture, it has limitations, and is

---

*The authors interviewed and filmed acupuncturists in Hong Kong, Japan, and the United States to learn more about its application to pain control.

merely an alternate method of reducing pain. Hypnosis may be viewed simply as increased suggestion. If your dentist tells you, "You're only going to feel a tiny prick," you're likely to accept that and feel less discomfort than if you were all set for a horrible, painful experience. Hypnosis works on the same principle. The patient's increased susceptibility to suggestion results in sensory and motor capacities being altered. The patient receives the suggestions, accepts them as facts, and acts accordingly.

Hypnotism may be a very dramatic way of producing anesthesia, and probably only a small percentage of people are even susceptible to complete hypnoanesthesia. But a good dentist employs some aspects of hypnosis every time he talks to you. The sound of his voice can calm you and relax you, suggesting to you that what you are about to have done is not unpleasant and is certainly beneficial.

Hypnodontics is not practical for *every* patient. It may involve a light trance, a deep trance, or waking hypnotic suggestion. Most of the desired effects can be reached in 5 to 10 minutes of the light trance, and it is effective in about 80% of cases. But local anesthetics in small amounts must also be used.

The deep trance is used where medication is not possible, and only about 20% of the population are susceptible to it. Post hypnotic suggestions are used to prolong the effects, to avoid a post-trance headache, or to prepare for the next visit.

Induction of moods and states of mind have been shown to alter consciousness, change blood pressure, and even decrease bleeding and salivation. But most dentists find it is too time consuming, and the results are still not predictable. There is also the danger of hallucinations and catalepsy, and it is clearly contraindicated for psychotics.

For certain dentally-related and emotionally based conditions like thumb sucking, nail biting, and bruxism, it may have additional application. But for most patients, it's simply an adjunct to conventional techniques which dentists prefer to use.

Research

A new army of healing scientists consisting of biological physicists, virologists, pharmacologists, microbiologists, bio-atomic engineers, and other hybrid specialists are rapidly emerging on the health scene. The National Institute of Dental Research, the research departments of dental schools and hospitals, and government financed programs are also engaged in intensive research studies to bring advances and improvements to dentistry.

When research perfects a commercially available decay control vaccine, and we can abort or eliminate periodontal problems, we will have eliminated 95% of all dental disease. Then, perhaps, the profession of dentistry will be eliminated much the same way that the blacksmith and the iceman have all but disappeared from the American scene.

12
Dental Consumerism and You

We Americans spend more than $100 billion a year for health care, which is the third largest industry in our country, employing about four and one-half million people. We *must not,* therefore, abrogate our roles in determining the quality of that care and the money we spend for it.

After all, *health care is a necessity.* You can put off buying a piano, taking a vacation, or replacing your living room rug. But if your face is all blown up with an impacted wisdom tooth and you're writhing in pain, the necessity for dental care is all too clear. We Americans are spending more than 8% of the Gross National Product on health care. Aren't we entitled to a say in how that "product" is dispensed to us and what it's going to cost us?

In today's inflation ridden marketplace, everyone wants to find a way to hold down the spiraling costs of health care and those horrendous bills that take such a big chunk out of our budgets. But you also want to be sure no one's cutting corners on you, that you're getting what you paid for, and that the quality doesn't suffer.

Private health care is not alone in escalating costs. The cost of government sponsored programs have been increasing even faster. The overall cost of private medical care went up about 14%,* but the two key government programs almost doubled. Medicaid went up 25% and Medicare went up 30%.

*According to 1975 figures.

Who is picking up that bill? *You* are! Therefore, you *must* become involved in the issues. How? First, become informed. Next, insist that your voice be heard. That's *consumerism* — the hottest *ism* in America today. You, the dental consumer, have that right. In fact, it is your obligation. If you don't like the way things are run, you can't complain unless:

1. You are informed on the issues.
2. You actively participate in the policy making decisions.

Until recent years, most buyers thought of themselves as individual purchasers. Each buyer dealt on an individual basis with an individual seller. As a result, *buyers remained a vast, unorganized, heterogeneous number of individual purchasers who had nothing in common.* If someone got stuck on a purchase, he could ask the seller to make good. But if the seller refused, what could he do?

Some stalwart foes of the rip-off, fired by indignation, frustration, and anger, "went further." They reported their grievance to the Better Business Bureau, the Chamber of Commerce, and maybe even a government agency. But the red tape and meager results often did *not* bring satisfaction. At most, the seller got off with a slap on the wrist or a small fine.

All that has changed. Buyers of any product or service, from a yacht to a yellow ribbon, are demanding and getting satisfaction. How? By organizing. Consumer groups, unions, and associations have sprung up all over our country at every level — city, state, and national. These groups are discovering that *consumers have rights, too,* and consumers need a "union" to look out for those rights, to protect them from abuses, and to punish offenders.

Untouched by all this consumerism have been "the learned professions." If a shopkeeper sold a defective product, he could be reprimanded. But a dentist? A physician? Never! Traditionally, they have been exempt from attention by consumer groups.

The thinking behind this was based on the absurd attitude that physicians, dentists, and lawyers were "above" that sort of thing. They were a breed apart whose high moral values and exemplary standards of behavior were never soiled by the flotsam and jetsam of the business world. A doctor was not interested in the marketplace and the crass world of commerce. He was dedicated to helping people. Money be damned!

Even today, despite scathing experiences in dental offices and medical offices, and despite the steady dehumanization of patients by disinterested, even incompetent hospital personnel, some people still cling to the image of their physician or dentist as a mini-God, incapable of soiling his hands with money. These patients remain implacable in their steadfast loyalty and awe of their dentists.

Nothing can hurt you, the consumer, more than this ridiculous, naive notion. *You are buying – yes, buying – a service from your dentist.* You are entitled to satisfaction

> **Dissatisfaction Gets Refunds**
>
> *At the Blanchard Valley Hospital in Findlay, Ohio, the customers are always right. The hospital guarantees the 40,000 patients treated annually good food, good nursing care, and other amenities. Justified complaints produce a refund. Should you settle for less?*

The American Dental Association spends *millions to lobby for the self-interest of their members: dentists.* Shouldn't you look out for yourself? The American Dental Association does many good things for consumers: they rate products, issue useful educational materials, and maintain standards for the profession of dentistry. But for the most part, they are looking out for the interests of dentists. This is, of course, consistent with any "union," whether it be the United Mine Workers, the Teamsters, or the American Association of University Professors. But who looks out for you? *Perhaps there should be a Patient's Union,* a separate and distinct branch of the consumer groups in America today. Better yet, the institution of a Federal Consumer Agency at the Cabinet level, complete with a Federal Data Bank of Consumer Information, might be a giant step forward.

This book attempts to raise your consciousness about some of these issues, to inform you, and perhaps even to move you to action. Consider how the American Dental Association is on *their* toes about any issue that can adversely affect dentists. They tax their members through dues, and they issue carefully constructed "recommendations" to their members. They lobby constantly for what they want. Their power is tremendous.

For example, a recent "Information Bulletin" of some months ago was sent to all their members. It alerted them and warned the dentists:

Deep federal intrusion into education;
dentists urged to act quickly — contact Senators.

If you act quickly, this week, you can bring your influence to bear on matters that affect your practice.

The bulletin went on to spell out, *point by point,* their objections to an upcoming bill HR5546, the Health Professions Educational Assistance Act. They urged every dentist to visit or send letters to their two Senators. "YOU MUST ACT TODAY" was boxed off in large letters. They warned against the passage of the bill, and concluded with *detailed instructions,* under a special heading titled "HOW TO SAY IT," which outlined 7 points for every dentist to cover.

That's the power of a lobby! Can you afford to have less power?

What Consumerism Means to You

Consumerism does *not* mean you should be out to "get" your dentist. Consumerism does *not* mean you should be suspicious, hostile, or constantly on guard against your dentist. The truth is that most dentists are decent, honorable men and women, highly trained, and deeply motivated to care about their patients. They *want* to give you satisfaction. And in most cases, they do.

But that doesn't mean that once you open wide, you should leave yourself wide open. You have rights, too. Many consumer organizations are recognizing that and formulating "A Dental Patient's Bill Of Rights." If you know what you're entitled to and understand the professional services you're buying, you don't abrogate those rights.

Today's patients are less likely to let their doctors make choices for them. Women are questioning the number of unnecessary hysterectomies and mastectomies that have been performed, and patients want a say in those matters which affect their bodies and their budgets. Today's patients are better informed about sophisticated techniques and scientific advancements. They read, watch television, and engage in "cocktail party debates" over medical and dental controversies. All of this has resulted in marked changes and altered relationships between patients and their doctors.

The emergence of the Public Policy Dentist demonstrates that dentists, too, have entered the field of consumerism. Ralph Nader calls them "the watchdogs of dentistry." Imagine a dentist who does *not treat* patients, but is concerned only with the broad issues of patient's rights, the quality of dental care, the distribution of dentists, dental insurance, health legislation, safety, drugs, and fees. These are all *issues to benefit you, the consumer.* Perhaps the day will come when dentists and patients will *not* be on different sides, but can join forces for the mutual benefit of each other.

Consumer Heroes and Consumer Zeroes

In the meantime, the Consumer Federation of America, our country's largest consumer organization, has issued a statement which features a list of CONSUMER HEROES AND CONSUMER ZEROES for the first session of the 94th Congress. These are the *legislators who consistently voted or failed to vote for the best interests of the consumer on at least 75% of the key issues.*

Heading the list of CONSUMER ZEROES in the Senate were:

James Buckley (N.Y.)   Lloyd Bentsen (Texas)
Robert Taft, Jr. (Ohio)   Harry F. Byrd (Va.)

In the House of Representatives, the CONSUMER ZEROES were:

Alaska:	Don Young	Conn.:	Ronald A. Sarasin
Ariz.:	Sam Steiger	Fla.:	Richard Kelly
	John Conlan	Ga.:	John J. Flynt, Jr.
Calif.:	Don H. Clausen		Larry McDonald
	Burt L. Talsott	Idaho:	George Hansen
	William M. Ketchum	Ill.:	Henry J. Hyde
	Del Clawson		George M. O'Brien
	Shirley Pettis	Iowa:	Charles E. Grassley
	Bob Wilson	Kansas:	Garner E. Shriver

La.:	W. Henson Moore	Okla.:	Theodore Risenhoover
Md.:	Robert E. Bauman		Glenn English
Mich.:	Garry Brown	Pa.:	Herman T. Schneebeli
	Edward Hutchinson		Albert W. Johnson
Minn.:	Tom Hagedorn	Tex.:	Robert Krueger
Mo.:	Gene Taylor	Va.:	J. Kenneth Robertson
Neb.:	Virginia Smith	Wisc.:	Robert W. Kasten, Jr.
Ohio:	Willis D. Gradison, Jr.		
	Donald D. Clansy		
	Thomas N. Kindness		

In total, 14 Senators and 64 members of the House of Representatives *failed to cast a single vote in the best interests of consumerism.* Here is the complete list:

CONSUMER ZEROES (Senators)

Zero percent – Senators who never voted for the consumer.

Arizona:	Fannin	North Carolina:	Helms
	Goldwater	North Dakota:	Young
Idaho:	McClure	Oklahoma:	Bartlett
Mississippi:	Eastland		Bellmon
Nebraska:	Curtis	South Carolina:	Thurmond
	Hruska	Utah:	Garn
Nevada:	Laxalt	Wyoming:	Hansen

CONSUMER ZEROES (Representatives)

Zero percent – House of Representatives Members who never voted for the consumer. (district no. in parentheses)

Alabama:	Edwards (1)	California:	Wilson (41)
	Dickinson (2)	(cont.)	Wilson (41)
Alaska:	Young (AL)		Burgener (43)
Arizona:	Rhodes (1)	Colorado:	Armstrong (5)
	Conlan (4)	Florida:	Kelly (5)
California:	Clausen (2)		Haley (8)
	Talcott (16)		Frey (9)
	Ketchum (18)	Georgia:	Landrum (9)
	Lagomarsino (19)		Stephens (10)
	Goldwater (20)	Idaho:	Symms (1)
	Rousselot (26)		Hansen (2)
	Pettis (37)	Illinois:	Crane (12)

CONSUMER ZEROES (Representatives)

Illinois:	O'Brien (17)	Ohio:	Devine (12)
(cont.)	Findley (20)	(cont.)	Wylie (15)
Indiana:	Myers (7)		Ashbrook (17)
Kansas:	Winn (3)	Oklahoma:	Risenhoover (2)
Louisiana:	Treen (3)		Jarmin (5)
	Moore (6)	Pennsylvania:	Shuster (9)
Maryland:	Bauman (1)		Goodling (19)
	Holt (4)	Tennessee:	Quillen (1)
	Byron (6)		Beard (6)
Michigan:	Esch (2)	Texas:	Archer (7)
	Brown (3)		Hightower (13)
	Hutchinson (4)		de la Garza (15)
	Cederberg (10)		Krueger (21)
Missouri:	Taylor (7)	Virginia:	Satterfield (3)
Nebraska:	McCollister (2)		Daniel, R. (4)
	Smith (3)		Daniel, D. (5)
New Mexico:	Runnels (2)		Butler (6)
New York:	Hastings (39)		Robinson (7)
North Carolina:	Broyhill (10)		Wampler (9)
Ohio:	Guyer (4)	Wisconsin:	Kasten (9)
	Brown (7)		

Carol Tucker Foreman, executive director of Consumer Federation of America, says:

We publish our list of Heroes and Zeroes to inform the American consumers about which of their elected representatives are truly concerned with their problems and which are continually selling out to the interests of big business.

Ms. Foreman obviously feels strongly about it. "Those on our Zero list," she says, "are pickpockets."

Fortunately, you can see there were several CONSUMER HEROES, too. 7 Senators and 57 Representatives scored 100% ratings. They were:

(7) CONSUMER HEROES (Senate)

Floyd K. Haskell (Colo.)
William D. Hathaway (Maine)
John Durkin & Thomas J. McIntyre (N. Hamp.)
Harrison A. Williams & Clifford P. Case (N.J.)
Richard S. Schweiker (Pa.)

(57) CONSUMER HEROES (House of Representatives)

House of Representatives — Perfect Record — 100%

California:	Moss (3)	New Jersey:	Howard (3)
	Burton, J. (5)		Maguire (7)
	Miller (7)		Roe (8)
	Dellums (8)		Minish (11)
	Edwards (10)	New York:	Downey (2)
	Waxman (24)		Ambro (3)
	Roybal (25)		Addabbo (7)
	Burke (28)		Rosenthal (8)
	Hawkins (29)		Scheuer (11)
Connecticut:	Cotter (1)		Chisholm (12)
	Moffett (6)		Holtzman (16)
Illinois:	Murphy (2)		Badillo (21)
	Yates (9)	Ohio:	Whalen (3)
Indiana:	Roush (4)		Carney (19)
Iowa:	Mezvinsky (1)		Stokes (21)
	Harkin (5)	Oregon:	Weaver (4)
Maryland:	Sarbanes (3)	Pennsylvania:	Green (3)
	Mitchell (7)		Edgar (7)
	Gude (8)		Rooney (15)
Mass.:	Boland (2)	Rhode Island:	St. Germain (1)
	Early (3)	Virginia:	Harris (8)
	Drinan (4)	West Virginia:	Hechler (4)
	Tsongas (5)	Wisconsin:	Baldus (3)
	Moakley (9)		Zablocki (4)
	Burke (11)		Reuss (5)
	Studds (12)		Obey (7)
Michigan:	Carr (6)		Cornell (8)
	Ford (15)		
Minnesota:	Nolan (6)		
	Oberstar (8)		

256 HOW TO SAVE YOUR TEETH AND YOUR MONEY

A number of Senators or Representatives *never voted against the consumer, but didn't score a perfect 100% due to absenteeism.* They were considered "Absent Advocates" by Ms. Foreman. Who were they?

Senators

Abraham Ribicoff (Conn.)
Adlai Stevenson (Ill.)
Birch Bayh (Ind.)
Edward Brooke (Mass.)
Lee Metcalf (Mont.)
James Abourezk (S.D.)

House of Representatives

Absent Advocates — House of Representatives: Those who never voted against the consumer but were absent one or more times.

Arizona:	Udall (2)	Missouri:	Clay (1)
California:	Burton, P. (6)		Sullivan (3)
	Stark (1)	New Jersey:	Floria (1)
	Wilson (31)		Thompson (4)
	Lloyd (35)		Helstoski (9)
	Van Deerlin (42)		Rodino (10)
Florida:	Pepper (14)		Daniels (14)
Illinois:	Metcalfe (1)	New York:	Solarz (13)
	Fary (5)		Richmond (14)
	Collins (7)		Koch (18)
	Rostenkowski (8)		Rangel (19)
	Mikva (10)		Abzug (20)
	Annunzio (11)		Bingham (22)
Indiana:	Brademas (3)		Ottinger (24)
Maryland:	Spellman (5)		McHugh (27)
Mass.:	Harrington (6)	Ohio:	Seiberling (14)
Michigan:	Conyers (1)		Vanik (22)
	Riegle (7)	Pennsylvania:	Mottl (23)
	Diggs (13)		Nix (2)
Minnesota:	Darth (4)	Rhode Island:	Ellberg (4)
	Fraser (5)	West Virginia:	Beard (2)
			Staggers (2)

Although elections in your state may have replaced some of your Senators or Representatives, and the tally for the second half of the

94th Congress is not yet in, you can still *check this list to see who is on your side.* You can also keep a sharp eye out to observe the voting record of newly elected Senators and Representatives, as the consumer bills continue to come up.

To stay on top of this issue, you can sent $1 to:

> CONSUMER FEDERATION OF AMERICA
> 10012 14th Street N.W.
> Washington, D.C. 20005

Of course, the issues your elected representatives voted on do not reflect specific *dental* issues. They cover a wide range of consumer concerns such as rising prices, food stamps, banking regulations, oil price decontrol, and many others. Nevertheless, if you've never taken part in consumer concerns, this could be an excellent introduction.

State and local consumer groups are also active in protecting your interests. You may decide to join such a group and introduce patient rights concerns into their programs.

In any case, whatever road you choose, if you've read this book you're bound to be a wise dental consumer and a more informed, more astute dental patient. The next time you pay your dentist a visit, you'll be armed with what you've learned and *you're bound to save yourself money.* You'll know what questions to ask, how to make wise choices, and how to keep costs down. You'll be your own dental consumer advocate, and you're likely to come off better.

Dr. Eva Kornblith, that 84 year old periodontist from New Jersey said:

> *I still have all my teeth and so should everybody else. After 52 years as a practicing periodontist, I am convinced that prevention is the most wonderful part of the profession.*

A good bit of that prevention can be done by you right in your own home. Then your dentist can follow up with professional care.

Dental consumerism is a brand new idea. Once you believe in it, read about it, and talk about it, you're likely to attract others who feel the way you do: *that dental patients have legitimate consumer concerns.*

Everyone has teeth and everyone has a wallet. Exercise your rights and you can save your teeth and your money!

Index

abscess, 24, 34, 62, 85, 86, 101
accident, 49, 53
acids, 50
acupuncture, 244
adjustments, 45, 71, 86, 98
advertising, 237-238
adult orthodontia, 46-48, 152-153
amalgam, 7, 64, 68, 82
American Dental Association, 62, 63, 66, 94, 97, 99, 120, 121, 126, 205, 225, 226, 228, 231, 233-234, 237, 250
American Medical Association, 79, 96, 237, 238
analgesia, 58, 101
anchor tooth, 46, 173
anesthesia, 31, 43, 49, 57, 58, 101, 167, 188, 244
angina, 42
apicoectomy, 158
appointments, 20, 30, 33, 197-198
aspirin, 58-59, 100
auxiliaries, 20-21, 31, 33, 234

baby teeth, 38-40, 224. *See also* primary teeth
behavior modification, 102
billing, 67-69, 199-200
biofeedback, 43
biopsy, 2, 189
bite, 47, 57, 82
bite plate, 43, 166

bleeding gums, 37, 51-53, 82, 162-163, 165
bone, 52, 165
bone transplant, 166, 213
bottle feeding, 130-131
braces, 151, 239. *See also* orthodontia
brackets, metal, 47
brackets, plastic, 47, 220, 239
breast feeding, 130-131
bridges, fixed, 13, 46, 49, 64, 68, 82, 113, 169, 170, 176-179
bridges, removable, 13, 68, 113, 169. *See also* partial dentures
bruxism, 106, 164
buck teeth, 47, 152, 219

calcium, 37
calculus, 163
cancer, 2, 18, 24, 25, 28, 188-189
canker sore, 36, 167
cap. *See* crown
Carter, President Jimmy, 121, 225
cavities, 15, 16, 93, 100, 105, 107, 229
checkup, 16, 33, 88, 89, 92, 166, 216
cheek, 36, 57
chemanesia, 188
chewing, 36, 46, 47, 82, 152
chewing gum, 50-51
choking, 105-106
clasp, 43-44, 51, 171
cleanliness, 30, 33
cleft palate, 187

259

260 INDEX

clinic, 18, 223
cold sore, 18, 36, 100, 167
composite resins, 82, 218-219
computers, 239-240
consultation, 17-18
consumer advocate, 65
Consumer Federation of America, 252, 254 257
Consumer Heroes, 252-256
consumer laws, 83-84
consumer organizations, 65, 66, 67, 249, 251, 252, 254, 257
consumer survey, 65-67
CONSUMER TIPS, 109-110, 124, 145, 154, 161, 168, 183-184, 191
Consumer Zeroes, 252-256
continuing education, 68, 233
cosmetic improvement, 47, 113, 146, 153, 173, 187, 216
credit, 226-227
crown, 51, 61, 67, 81, 82, 90, 130, 164, 179-182, 216
curettage, 82, 115, 165, 166
cut rate dentistry, 40, 77-79
cyst, 187

decay, 16, 38
deciduous, 38. *See also* baby teeth
Denholtz Muscle Anchorage Appliance, 148
dental floss, 97-98, 164, 166
dental nurses, 121, 234-235
dental school clinics, 70-71
dental schools, 71-74, 229
dentifrices. *See* toothpaste
denture adhesives, 98-99, 173, 178
denture cleaners, 99, 173
denture repairs, 86
dentures, 44-45, 51, 61, 64, 65, 66, 71, 76, 78, 79, 85, 91, 92, 99, 105, 113, 164, 169, 172-176, 222, 242
denturism, 76
diagnosis, 24, 28
diastema, 218
diet, 41, 56, 60, 144
digestion, 41, 97
disclosing tablets, 164, 166, 195
drifting, 38, 39, 143, 177

edentulous, 78, 169
electric toothbrush, 93-94

emergency, 21-22, 30, 53, 76, 100-101, 187
enamel, 50, 54-55
endodontia, 78, 126, 155-161
endodontist, 50, 155
equilibration, 43
eruption, 38, 56
estimate, 11, 26, 28
examination, 13
exodontia, 126, 185-191
exodontist, 185
extraction mills, 14-15, 28, 69, 78, 174
extractions, 14, 15, 29, 33, 38, 39, 40-41, 46, 48, 64, 78, 82, 85, 90, 113, 143, 148-150, 174-176, 185, 190

false teeth, 42, 78, 169
fear, 58, 101-102, 128-129, 203
fees, 10-11, 25, 26, 32, 45, 61-91, 146-147, 151-152, 157, 158, 166
fiber optics, 240-241
fillings, 61, 64, 65, 71, 81, 82, 88, 101, 113, 141, 142, 164, 182
fluoride, 16, 54-56, 70, 94, 130, 132-139, 170-171, 178, 181, 193, 194, 211, 214, 216, 217, 220
forensic dentistry, 243-244
fractured jaw, 187
fraud, 68, 83, 95, 225, 230, 233

gas, 56
gingivectomy, 64, 88, 166
gingivitis, 52, 165
gingivoplasty, 166
gold inlay, 64, 82
government clinic, 75-76
group practice, 20, 31, 69-70, 224
gums, 14, 16, 70, 85, 88, 98, 129, 130, 131

halitosis, 96, 97, 162
hay rake, 139
headaches, 28, 42-43, 57, 58, 106-107
head caps, 147
Health Maintenance Organization (HMO), 79-81
history, 13, 27, 33
hormones, 35, 37, 144, 165
hospitalization, 113
hygiene, 46, 56, 60, 82, 92, 98, 144
hygienist, 17, 20, 21, 31, 65, 200, 234

INDEX

hypersensitivity, 95
hypnodontics, 245-246
hypnosis, 102

immediate dentures, 85, 173
impactions, 45, 185, 218-219
implants, 189-190, 213-214, 215, 242
incompetency, 69, 81, 82, 193, 230
infection, 39, 45, 97
inflammation, 52
injuries, 107
insurance, 8, 12-13, 84, 89, 111-124, 146, 186, 195-196, 205-206
    deductible limitations and exclusions, 113
    Delta plans, 118-120, 121
    dual coverage, 116
    insurance forms, 114-117, 118
    maximizing benefits, 114
    medical insurance, 113
    table of allowances, 113
    third party payments, 112, 117
    usual, customary and reasonable (UCR), 111, 113
interceptive orthodontics, 147-148
irrigating devices, 95-96

jacket. *See* crown
jaw bone, 38, 46, 58, 59, 87, 169, 173, 240
jaw joint, 13, 81
junk food, 50, 144

laboratory, 44, 67
laboratory technician, 44, 67
lantern jaw, 186
lasers, 35
lead bib, 25, 32, 66, 86
licenses, 23, 231-233
lip, 36, 57, 100, 167
loose teeth, 52, 162-164

malocclusion, 42, 47, 139, 146, 147, 152
malpractice insurance, 122-123
mandible, 186
maxillo-facial surgeon, 185
medicaid, 69, 115, 248
medical problems, 28, 40-42, 97
mobile clinics, 230
motivation, 107-108, 206

mouth breathing, 164, 223
mouth protectors, 100
mouth rehabilitation, 26, 89, 90, 211
mouthwash, 16, 96-97, 100, 105, 189
myofunctional therapy, 140
myths, 34-60, 129, 152-153

Nader, Ralph, 65, 252
National Health Insurance, 120-122, 225
National Institute of Dental Research, 105, 247
needle, 31-32, 33, 56
nerve, 49
night brace, 147
nitrous oxide, 58
nursing bottle, 131
nursing bottle syndrome, 140-141
nutrition, 41, 92, 102, 104, 129

occlusion, 13, 107
oral hygiene, 16
oral surgeon, 185, 187
oral surgery, 186
orthodontia, 29, 38, 46-48, 76, 78, 113, 125, 126, 146-154, 217, 223
orthodontist, 70, 126, 146, 220
osteoplasty, 166
overdenture, 176

pacifiers, 139-140
pain, 9-10, 48-50, 57, 61, 82, 84, 85, 87, 88, 102, 128, 151, 155, 167, 219
palate, 13
Panorex X ray, 68, 87, 212
partial denture, 9, 43-44, 51, 64, 79, 85, 87, 88, 90, 170-171
patient profile, 208-209
payment plan, 11-12
pedodontia, 126, 127-145
pedodontist, 40, 70, 128
peer review, 69, 230
periodontia, 76, 78, 82, 113, 126, 157, 162-168
periodontist, 52, 70, 162
periodontitis, 52, 165
permanent teeth, 39, 46, 142
personality, of dentist, 16-17, 29
pharmacy, 95, 195, 224
pit and fissure sealants, 107

INDEX

plates. *See* dentures
plastic brackets. *See* brackets
plastic surgery, 173, 187
plaque, 16, 52, 65, 94, 163
pockets, 14, 52, 163, 240
polyps, 189
porcelain crown, 9, 63, 64, 181, 215
positioner, 151
post, 213
precision attachment, 171
pregnancy, 24, 37-38
premedication, 101
preventive dentistry, 15-16, 80
primary teeth 38, 131-132. *See also* baby teeth
private interest clinic, 77
prognosis, 7
prophylaxis, 21, 64, 65, 113, 115, 216
prosthodontia, 126, 169-184
prosthodontist, 169, 187
psychological aspects, 8, 29, 47, 90, 102, 128, 152, 172, 215
public policy dentist, 227, 252
pulp, 49
pulp cap, 15, 159
pulpotomy, 142-143
pus, 52
pyorrhea, 51-53, 165

quality, 65, 66, 69, 81-82

referrals, 19, 207
reimplantation, 53
reline, 45, 86, 174
reline kit, 44, 99
removable appliances, 47. *See also* partial denture
research, 246-247
retainer, 151
reverse swallowing, 140
root, 53, 141
root canal, 14, 15, 29, 49-50, 64, 65, 71, 88, 89, 114, 155-161, 213, 240
rubber dam, 82

saliva test, 241
Sargenti, 127, 159-160
sex, 7, 172
Sexton-Shealy Clinic, 66, 78
shot. *See* anesthesia or needle

silver filling. *See* amalgam
sinus, 28, 87, 100
smile, 47, 90
smoking, 189, 211
socket, 53-54
sonar devices, 240
sore spots, 44, 82, 99
space maintainer, 39, 143
specialist, 126-127
speech, 39, 152, 187
sphygmomanometer, 2
State Board examinations, 23, 227-228, 231
stimudents, 98
stress, 43
study models, 13, 27, 88, 149, 153, 212
sugar, 50, 96, 103-105
supernumerary teeth, 59
surfaces of tooth, 61-62
surgery, 43, 113, 165-166, 167

tartar, 163
taste, 173
team dentistry, 235
teenagers, 143-144
teething, 131
temporomandibular joint (TMJ), 42-43, 152, 177, 187, 212
thumb sucking, 139
tongue, 13
tongue thrusting, 131, 140
toothache, 16, 28, 35, 48-49, 58, 59, 76, 85, 100, 141, 142, 222. *See also* pain
tooth bank, 241
toothbrushes, 16, 50, 52, 56, 76, 93, 99, 141, 195, 196
tooth fairy, 60
toothpaste, 56, 94-95, 141, 195
toothpicks, 98
treatment, 14-15
treatment plan, 6, 26, 32
trench mouth, 167
tumors, 14

unions, 77, 112, 226

vaccines, 243
Vincent's Infection, 167
visual aids, 18
vitamins, 35, 102-103

whiskey, 58-59
wisdom tooth, 29, 45-46, 64, 82, 143, 185, 218
women in dentistry, 235-236

X rays, 13, 15, 19, 23-25, 27, 31, 32, 64, 68, 70, 71, 85, 86, 87, 88, 113, 117, 130, 142, 149, 212, 239

GIVE YOUR DENTIST A DENTAL CHECKUP.
(If he scores 4 or more, consider changing dentists.)

1. ☐ YOUR DENTIST DOES NOT TAKE X RAYS. (Score 1 point.)
2. ☐ YOUR DENTIST DOES TAKE X RAYS, BUT HE HOLDS THEM WITH HIS OWN FINGER. (Score 1 point.)
3. ☐ YOUR DENTIST TAKES X RAYS, BUT ASKS YOU, THE PATIENT, TO HOLD THE FILM WITH YOUR FINGER. (Score ½ point.)
4. ☐ YOUR DENTIST TAKES X RAYS, BUT DOES NOT DRAPE A PROTECTIVE LEAD BIB OVER YOUR BODY. (Score ½ point.)
5. ☐ YOUR DENTIST DOES NOT GIVE A DETAILED EXPLANATION OF HIS FEES BEFORE WORK IS STARTED. (Score 1 point.)
6. ☐ YOUR DENTIST CHARGES UNUSUALLY HIGH OR UNUSUALLY LOW FEES. (Score ½ point.)
7. ☐ YOUR DENTIST SUGGESTS AN EXPENSIVE TREATMENT PLAN. YOU ARE UNDECIDED, CONFUSED, AND WISH TO GET ANOTHER OPINION. YOUR DENTIST IS HOSTILE, RESENTFUL AND UNCOOPERATIVE. (Score 1 point.)
8. ☐ YOUR DENTIST DOES NOT TAKE A MEDICAL-DENTAL HISTORY AT YOUR INITIAL VISIT. (Score 1 point.)
9. ☐ YOUR DENTIST ADVISES YOU THAT YOUR HEADACHES, BACKACHES, SINUSITIS, DIABETES, ARTHRITIS, AND FATIGUE ARE COMING FROM YOUR INFECTED TEETH, AND YOU SHOULD HAVE THEM ALL REMOVED. (Score this 4 points and leave the office.)
10. ☐ YOUR DENTIST ADVISES YOU TO HAVE ONE OR MORE TEETH EXTRACTED WITHOUT TRYING TO SAVE THEM. (Don't include wisdom teeth or teeth to be removed for orthodontic purposes. Score 1 point.)
11. ☐ YOUR DENTIST DOES NOT SEE YOU AS A PERSON, BUT AS A TOOTH. (Score ½ point.)
12. ☐ YOUR DENTIST FREQUENTLY KEEPS YOU WAITING FOR AN HOUR, AND IS INCONSIDERATE OF YOUR TIME. (Score ½ point.)
13. ☐ YOUR DENTIST'S OFFICE IS UNCLEAN AND SHABBY. (Score ½ point.)
14. ☐ YOUR DENTIST DOES NOT EMPLOY ANY DENTAL ASSISTANT OR AUXILIARY PERSONNEL. (Score ½ point.)
15. ☐ YOUR DENTIST DOES NOT USE DISPOSABLE NEEDLES. (Score 1 point.)

☐ TOTAL SCORE

GIVE YOUR DENTIST A DENTAL CHECKUP.
(If he scores 4 or more, consider changing dentists.)

1. ☐ YOUR DENTIST DOES NOT TAKE X RAYS. (Score 1 point.)
2. ☐ YOUR DENTIST DOES TAKE X RAYS, BUT HE HOLDS THEM WITH HIS OWN FINGER. (Score 1 point.)
3. ☐ YOUR DENTIST TAKES X RAYS, BUT ASKS YOU, THE PATIENT, TO HOLD THE FILM WITH YOUR FINGER. (Score ½ point.)
4. ☐ YOUR DENTIST TAKES X RAYS, BUT DOES NOT DRAPE A PROTECTIVE LEAD BIB OVER YOUR BODY. (Score ½ point.)
5. ☐ YOUR DENTIST DOES NOT GIVE A DETAILED EXPLANATION OF HIS FEES BEFORE WORK IS STARTED. (Score 1 point.)
6. ☐ YOUR DENTIST CHARGES UNUSUALLY HIGH OR UNUSUALLY LOW FEES. (Score ½ point.)
7. ☐ YOUR DENTIST SUGGESTS AN EXPENSIVE TREATMENT PLAN. YOU ARE UNDECIDED, CONFUSED, AND WISH TO GET ANOTHER OPINION. YOUR DENTIST IS HOSTILE, RESENTFUL AND UNCOOPERATIVE. (Score 1 point.)
8. ☐ YOUR DENTIST DOES NOT TAKE A MEDICAL-DENTAL HISTORY AT YOUR INITIAL VISIT. (Score 1 point.)
9. ☐ YOUR DENTIST ADVISES YOU THAT YOUR HEADACHES, BACKACHES, SINUSITIS, DIABETES, ARTHRITIS, AND FATIGUE ARE COMING FROM YOUR INFECTED TEETH, AND YOU SHOULD HAVE THEM ALL REMOVED. (Score this 4 points and leave the office.)
10. ☐ YOUR DENTIST ADVISES YOU TO HAVE ONE OR MORE TEETH EXTRACTED WITHOUT TRYING TO SAVE THEM. (Don't include wisdom teeth or teeth to be removed for orthodontic purposes. Score 1 point.)
11. ☐ YOUR DENTIST DOES NOT SEE YOU AS A PERSON, BUT AS A TOOTH. (Score ½ point.)
12. ☐ YOUR DENTIST FREQUENTLY KEEPS YOU WAITING FOR AN HOUR, AND IS INCONSIDERATE OF YOUR TIME. (Score ½ point.)
13. ☐ YOUR DENTIST'S OFFICE IS UNCLEAN AND SHABBY. (Score ½ point.)
14. ☐ YOUR DENTIST DOES NOT EMPLOY ANY DENTAL ASSISTANT OR AUXILIARY PERSONNEL. (Score ½ point.)
15. ☐ YOUR DENTIST DOES NOT USE DISPOSABLE NEEDLES. (Score 1 point.)

☐ TOTAL SCORE

GIVE YOUR DENTIST A DENTAL CHECKUP.
(If he scores 4 or more, consider changing dentists.)

1. ☐ YOUR DENTIST DOES NOT TAKE X RAYS. (Score 1 point.)
2. ☐ YOUR DENTIST DOES TAKE X RAYS, BUT HE HOLDS THEM WITH HIS OWN FINGER. (Score 1 point.)
3. ☐ YOUR DENTIST TAKES X RAYS, BUT ASKS YOU, THE PATIENT, TO HOLD THE FILM WITH YOUR FINGER. (Score ½ point.)
4. ☐ YOUR DENTIST TAKES X RAYS, BUT DOES NOT DRAPE A PROTECTIVE LEAD BIB OVER YOUR BODY. (Score ½ point.)
5. ☐ YOUR DENTIST DOES NOT GIVE A DETAILED EXPLANATION OF HIS FEES BEFORE WORK IS STARTED. (Score 1 point.)
6. ☐ YOUR DENTIST CHARGES UNUSUALLY HIGH OR UNUSUALLY LOW FEES. (Score ½ point.)
7. ☐ YOUR DENTIST SUGGESTS AN EXPENSIVE TREATMENT PLAN. YOU ARE UNDECIDED, CONFUSED, AND WISH TO GET ANOTHER OPINION. YOUR DENTIST IS HOSTILE, RESENTFUL AND UNCOOPERATIVE. (Score 1 point.)
8. ☐ YOUR DENTIST DOES NOT TAKE A MEDICAL-DENTAL HISTORY AT YOUR INITIAL VISIT. (Score 1 point.)
9. ☐ YOUR DENTIST ADVISES YOU THAT YOUR HEADACHES, BACKACHES, SINUSITIS, DIABETES, ARTHRITIS, AND FATIGUE ARE COMING FROM YOUR INFECTED TEETH, AND YOU SHOULD HAVE THEM ALL REMOVED. (Score this 4 points and leave the office.)
10. ☐ YOUR DENTIST ADVISES YOU TO HAVE ONE OR MORE TEETH EXTRACTED WITHOUT TRYING TO SAVE THEM. (Don't include wisdom teeth or teeth to be removed for orthodontic purposes. Score 1 point.)
11. ☐ YOUR DENTIST DOES NOT SEE YOU AS A PERSON, BUT AS A TOOTH. (Score ½ point.)
12. ☐ YOUR DENTIST FREQUENTLY KEEPS YOU WAITING FOR AN HOUR, AND IS INCONSIDERATE OF YOUR TIME. (Score ½ point.)
13. ☐ YOUR DENTIST'S OFFICE IS UNCLEAN AND SHABBY. (Score ½ point.)
14. ☐ YOUR DENTIST DOES NOT EMPLOY ANY DENTAL ASSISTANT OR AUXILIARY PERSONNEL. (Score ½ point.)
15. ☐ YOUR DENTIST DOES NOT USE DISPOSABLE NEEDLES. (Score 1 point.)

☐ TOTAL SCORE

GIVE YOUR DENTIST A DENTAL CHECKUP.
(If he scores 4 or more, consider changing dentists.)

1. ☐ YOUR DENTIST DOES NOT TAKE X RAYS. (Score 1 point.)
2. ☐ YOUR DENTIST DOES TAKE X RAYS, BUT HE HOLDS THEM WITH HIS OWN FINGER. (Score 1 point.)
3. ☐ YOUR DENTIST TAKES X RAYS, BUT ASKS YOU, THE PATIENT, TO HOLD THE FILM WITH YOUR FINGER. (Score ½ point.)
4. ☐ YOUR DENTIST TAKES X RAYS, BUT DOES NOT DRAPE A PROTECTIVE LEAD BIB OVER YOUR BODY. (Score ½ point.)
5. ☐ YOUR DENTIST DOES NOT GIVE A DETAILED EXPLANATION OF HIS FEES BEFORE WORK IS STARTED. (Score 1 point.)
6. ☐ YOUR DENTIST CHARGES UNUSUALLY HIGH OR UNUSUALLY LOW FEES. (Score ½ point.)
7. ☐ YOUR DENTIST SUGGESTS AN EXPENSIVE TREATMENT PLAN. YOU ARE UNDECIDED, CONFUSED, AND WISH TO GET ANOTHER OPINION. YOUR DENTIST IS HOSTILE, RESENTFUL AND UNCOOPERATIVE. (Score 1 point.)
8. ☐ YOUR DENTIST DOES NOT TAKE A MEDICAL-DENTAL HISTORY AT YOUR INITIAL VISIT. (Score 1 point.)
9. ☐ YOUR DENTIST ADVISES YOU THAT YOUR HEADACHES, BACKACHES, SINUSITIS, DIABETES, ARTHRITIS, AND FATIGUE ARE COMING FROM YOUR INFECTED TEETH, AND YOU SHOULD HAVE THEM ALL REMOVED. (Score this 4 points and leave the office.)
10. ☐ YOUR DENTIST ADVISES YOU TO HAVE ONE OR MORE TEETH EXTRACTED WITHOUT TRYING TO SAVE THEM. (Don't include wisdom teeth or teeth to be removed for orthodontic purposes. Score 1 point.)
11. ☐ YOUR DENTIST DOES NOT SEE YOU AS A PERSON, BUT AS A TOOTH. (Score ½ point.)
12. ☐ YOUR DENTIST FREQUENTLY KEEPS YOU WAITING FOR AN HOUR, AND IS INCONSIDERATE OF YOUR TIME. (Score ½ point.)
13. ☐ YOUR DENTIST'S OFFICE IS UNCLEAN AND SHABBY. (Score ½ point.)
14. ☐ YOUR DENTIST DOES NOT EMPLOY ANY DENTAL ASSISTANT OR AUXILIARY PERSONNEL. (Score ½ point.)
15. ☐ YOUR DENTIST DOES NOT USE DISPOSABLE NEEDLES. (Score 1 point.)

☐ TOTAL SCORE